Tales of a Sacred Prostitute

Revelations of How Sexual Energy Heals

Selena Truth

authorHOUSE®

AuthorHouse™
1663 Liberty Drive, Suite 200
Bloomington, IN 47403
www.authorhouse.com
Phone: 1-800-839-8640

First published by AuthorHouse 4/3/2009

ISBN: 978-1-4389-2679-7 (sc)

Printed in the United States of America
Bloomington, Indiana

Dedicated to Deborah Jeane Palfrey,
the "D.C. Madam"
who hung herself rather than go to prison.

She could have been me.

Table of Contents

Foreword

This is a tale of sexual excess and redemption. Not repentance, but a reclaiming of the healing and spiritual expansion that sexuality can catalyze.

Thousands of years ago, when the goddess was still worshipped, her priestesses used sexuality as part of their rites. With the advent of the patriarchy, sexuality was laden with shame and guilt. The split between the body and spirit, the feminine and the masculine, and earth and heaven began. The sacred prostitute was lost. The story of this is well told in <u>When God Was a Woman</u> by Merlin Stone.

Now the sacred prostitute is returning. Women and men are waking up, remembering the old ways. Kenneth Ray Stubbs' book <u>Women of the Light</u> describes many modern-day sacred prostitutes. When I read it, something stirred in me. I knew that I was destined to become a sacred prostitute myself.

I came into this life blessed with a powerful sexuality, with no idea of how to use it. Through blunders and pain, I slowly learned how to channel this gift. This was my path. I hope it serves you well.

I am no longer the person who is described in these pages. My days of being a sacred prostitute are mostly over now, at least in the form that I describe here. I do my priestess work differently -- but that will be the next book.

Most people think of the prostitute as a victim. The most visible prostitute is the streetwalker. She lives a dangerous life, and often experiences violence and abuse. This is the image of a prostitute in this culture, and it is how they are portrayed in movies and books.

However, there are many more sex workers who are not as visible. They are off the streets, safer although still not completely. There is always the possibility of a violent client or an undercover police officer walking through the door.

Most of the women and men that I have encountered in this business are not victims. They are people who freely choose this occupation. Often highly educated, they enjoy the work and the freedom it brings.

Who is to say what sacred prostitution is? To me, it is an individual path. There is no prescribed way to be a sacred prostitute. As long as the prostitute is choosing freely to do this work, then I support her or him to find the right way. I do not support any coerced kind of prostitution whatsoever.

Even though I no longer work in this way, I know that it is important to tell this story. We are on the verge of a new way of being, a way that honors the sacredness and healing powers of sexuality. If I can inspire others to remember, then that phase of my life will truly be complete. The legacy will continue.

I call to healers, and those in need of healing. Maybe including sexual energy in your process will serve you. It is a powerful force, a catalyst that brings issues to the surface that can then be addressed. Ignoring it means that a large part of the self is ignored.

I call to sex workers who have not explored the idea of the sacred prostitute. Perhaps this will inspire you to have the courage to bring more healing and spirituality into your work. Even if your clients don't expect it, you can bring this attitude to the work in a subtle fashion. People might not know why they are so drawn to you, but it will increase your business while you give something far greater than anything anticipated.

I call to other sacred prostitutes. I salute your courage to do this work in a time of such disapproval.

I call to those who are merely curious. I hope that these stories will engender a different attitude about sexuality and prostitution and the position they occupy in society. Rather than being something reviled and outlawed, sacred prostitution deserves to be honored and respected. As the attitudes of people change, then perhaps the laws that hamper the free flow of the sacred prostitute will change as well.

My spiritual path is Tantra, a branch of yoga that uses sexual energy as a pathway to the divine. Tantra includes many Sanskrit terms, which I have used throughout this book. If you come to an unfamiliar word, check the glossary for its definition.

All the stories in this book are true. I have changed the names, including my own, for privacy reasons. Someday perhaps that will not be necessary, when we truly embrace the concept of the sacred prostitute. Until then, I still wear the mask.

Acknowledgements

First, I want to thank Lisa Powers. Without her, this book would never have been written. She spent many weekends here at my mountain home, upstairs writing her book in my temple as I sat at my desk writing mine. As I finished a piece, I would bring it to her and she would edit it. I learned so much about writing from her, and we had a lot of fun together as well. Her presence and support kept me writing instead of avoiding it. I am deeply grateful.

Thanks to Kenneth Ray Stubbs for publishing <u>Women of the Light</u>, which inspired me to take this journey in the first place. His kindness in reading this book and giving feedback and encouragement was very valuable.

"Karen" provided me with a beautiful introduction to doing sensual massage, and became a dear friend. I appreciate how easy she made my transition in to sex work. She also read an early version of the book and gave valuable comments that helped shape it into what it is now.

I am grateful to "Jay" for the fun partnership that we enjoyed, both in the sensual massage business and later in our relationship. When my computer was stolen as I was writing this book, he bought me another one so I could keep on writing. He supported me in countless ways, and kept me laughing.

All the women with whom I worked during those years were wonderful. Their sense of humor and sense of the sacred made it such a fun journey. Sex workers are some of the most wild and exciting women I know.

I am very appreciative of all the wonderful men that I encountered as clients while doing this work. It was very enlightening to have such a wide experience of men's sexuality, and vastly rewarding on many levels to connect with so many generous, loving and respectful men. I learned how much men want to be received, even while in a role that makes them the receiver.

I thank "Peter" for being such solid support for so many years, for his role in opening me up to a deeper connection with Spirit, and for all the silly laughs we share. He is a dear companion in this life and I am blessed to be his friend.

Finally, I am grateful to "Adam" for motivating me to publish the book once it was finished. If it were not for him, I never would have put it out. I give deep thanks to him for his patience, wisdom, presence and juicy love. It is inspiring me to heal and blossom once again.

1 - The Gateway

Good Girl Goes Bad (In a Very Good Way)
2008 (age 54)

I am an innocent-looking woman. I rarely wear makeup or heels, or even dress up for that matter. My bright blue eyes are full of life, and meet other people's eyes with ease. My long thick hair is dyed a honey brown – a concession to the work I do. If I had my way, I'd leave it its natural darker brown with silver streaks, but I'm afraid that it might affect my income. Men seem to value youth in my profession, and I'm pushing the edge of acceptability. In another concession, I lie about my age to my clients. When I first started the work I was forty-five, but I said that I was thirty-eight. Now I'm fifty-four, and I vaguely say that I'm in my forties. I have such a youthful appearance that often men are surprised that I'm even as old as I say.

I don't look like the stereotype of a prostitute, yet technically that is what I have done for the last nine years. I have joined the small but growing ranks of the sacred prostitute. I do this work as a calling. It is holy work to me. I have plenty of other options for income. This is my choice.

When I was a girl I never planned that this is what I would do. I was raised with the same prejudices about prostitution that most people have. When I was eighteen, I went to a conservative women's college. To get a little extra spending money, I applied for a job as a nude model for the art department there. My parents had to sign to allow me to do this, and my father refused. "You might as well be a prostitute," he said scornfully.

Yet despite my wholesome looks and conservative upbringing, I somehow made my way into this work. It was a gradual process, even though the roots of the wildness in me were there from the beginning. It was one thing to be wild in my personal life, but another thing entirely to bring my sexuality into my work. It was like breaking the last taboo.

I eventually completed ten years of college, first getting a bachelor's degree in psychology and sociology, then going back to take sciences in order to go to four years of college in a field of natural health. I finished that training, and worked in the health professions for several years before making the transition into sex work.

How did a woman raised in the conservative South go from a health professional to a sacred prostitute? Here are some glimpses of my process.

Initiation
2005 (age 51)

"Wow," he said. "I don't think this has happened before."

His legs had started twitching and jumping with kundalini *(life force)* energy almost as soon as I started touching him.

"Looks like we're in for a wild ride today. Would you like to turn over?"

Once he was on his back I sat on the table between his legs and began slowly caressing him. I took my time, stroking each body part before gently spreading the sensations out to his whole body.

He ignited quickly. His cock pulsated, but he controlled his ejaculation. His body writhed on the table as he softly moaned.

"Slow down, slow down!" he said urgently.

Instantly I stopped the motion of my hand on his lingam *(penis).* I encouraged him to breathe the energy up his spine to his heart and hold it there. We paused, motionless.

As he exhaled, I began stroking him leisurely again. I slowly built his arousal, until he asked me to stop.

I directed him to breathe up into his heart. We repeated this again and again. As the energy got larger, I coached him to breathe it up to his third eye, the energy center in the fore-head.

"Bring the energy into your third eye. Put the tip of your tongue to the roof of your mouth to direct it there. Look up and inward towards the center of your forehead."

He followed my instructions, and I could see his eyelids flut-ter.

The next time he needed to pause, I told him to bring the energy all the way up to the crown.

"Imagine the top of your head is like a funnel, opening up to the heavens. Feel the connection with the spirit world through your crown."

I could feel my own crown open as he held the energy in his. Words began to come through me, without conscious thought.

"You're at the gateway here. You can enter the other realms now if you choose. Do you want to step through the gate-way?"

"Yes," he gasped.

Light filled me. It poured through, expanding until I became a huge column of light from my root to my crown. I continued to pleasure him, but it was the least of what was happening. The energy continued to grow and I began toning, letting sound move through me. The sounds got louder and louder.

His eyes widened in wonder as his body trembled and shook dramatically.

"I'm going to come!" he cried.

He began to ejaculate. I continued to stroke his lingam, still making sounds as the energy poured through me. He groaned in pleasure.

As he grew still, I began to slow myself down. I sat there quietly, still holding his penis in my hand.

"This was an initiation," I said to him. "This has shown you the pathway to the other realms. You can go there again now."

"The ecstasy was so big that I could barely stand it," he said.

"That's why you ejaculated, so you could get rid of the energy. You'll learn to keep going with it as you practice more. I teach people to tolerate ecstasy."

Opening
2006 (age 52)

Sean was a young man, with soulful dark eyes. He said that he had seen me once before although I did not remember him.

"Last time was so amazing," he said. "You told me there was a lot more. I want to find out what that is."

"That sounds great! " I said. "Please lie face down on the table."

After he made himself comfortable, I picked up my brass Tibetan singing bowl. I walked to the head of the table, and began an invocation.

"As I ring the bowl, come into this moment." I struck the bowl with the wooden ringer and beautiful clear tones filled the room, joining the sounds of the fountain on the altar nearby and the soft exotic music.

"Let all cares and concerns drop away." I rang the bowl again.

"Let the sounds bring you to higher realms." A third chime rang out. As the tones began to fade, I moved the bowl over his spine down to his root chakra (*energy center at the perineum*) to clear his energy.

"I wonder what I did with him? I wonder where we'll go today?" I thought to myself. I don't even try to remember people until I've seen them a couple of times, or I would be too cluttered with details. It's awkward sometimes when they have had an experience with such impact and I don't even remember them.

"Did you have anything in mind?" I asked him. "Or do you just want to see where it goes?"

"Let's just see where it goes," he said.

"Oh, good, now I can relax and forget about what might have happened last time," I thought.

I began lightly stroking his naked body, enjoying the curves of the muscles. His body was toned and fit, and I appreciated the beauty of it without being drawn to it sexually. I slowly moved up and down the length of him. Ever so often, I caressed his hair tenderly. I watched his body begin to relax.

I began to brush his inner thighs occasionally, as I passed them on the way up or down his body. I touched them just enough to get his attention, but not enough to make him fixate there yet.

Slowly and gradually, I caressed his testicles as I stroked the rest of his body. His pelvis began to move slightly as he became more aroused.

"It's time to work with his chakras now," I thought to myself. "His kundalini is starting to move."

My right hand stopped at his root chakra, and I touched him lightly with my middle fingertip on his perineum. I began to direct energy down my arm and through my hand into his root and up his spine. It felt like subtle tickles.

My left hand glided up his spine a few times, encouraging the kundalini to move, showing it the pathway. Then my hand rested at his sacrum to activate his second chakra. Consciously connecting my two hands, I transmitted from my right hand to my left, which was moving in small circles over his sacrum. I could feel his heat building. I began tapping gently on his perineum, with more urgency.

The movements of his pelvis began to get bigger and more dramatic. I watched as he writhed on the table.

"Time to start moving it upward," I thought to myself. "It has built enough now."

Several times I lightly slid my left hand from his sacrum to his heart chakra in the back, between his shoulder blades. I imagined the flow from his root to his heart. I had to visualize it at first, knowing that energy follows visualization and will. I was content to just begin the process of opening of the chakras, since I knew that I would do more when he turned over.

With my left hand, I moved from his heart over the top of his head. I rested the tip of my middle finger on his third eye at the center of his forehead, connecting to the fingertip of my right hand at his perineum. I paused there for a moment, feeling a small clear stream moving up through his body between my fingertips. Both my arms felt activated with energy.

His crown chakra was next. I lightly moved my left hand to the top of his head, surrounded it with my fingertips and magnetized a connection with my right hand at his root.

To complete my work on his back, I stroked the length of his body gently a few times. My hands came to rest on his sacrum and his heart. I paused, allowing him to absorb the quietness of the moment.

"Would you like to turn over?"

Slowly his body began to move as he came out of his trance enough to turn to his back. His lingam was erect and twitching slightly. He opened his eyes briefly.

"That was wonderful," he murmured.

"I'm so glad. There's more to come. Now that we've awakened the kundalini, we can use it. Would you like to know how?"

"Yes, I really want to learn."

"Once the kundalini is energized, you can direct it throughout your body. Imagine that there is a large tube going through the center of your body. It starts here," I touched his perineum. "And it goes all the way up to here." I touched the top of his head with my other hand.

"This is the channel for the flow of energy. Use a deep fast inhale to draw it up that channel, just like you are sucking something up a straw, and visualize it moving to wherever you'd like. Then hold your breath at the top of the inhalation for as long as you can. Understand?'

"Yes," he replied.

"Now, the art is in the timing. Do it too soon, and you'll never build any pleasure, because it makes it less intense when you spread it out. It's a way to delay ejaculation if you want to do that. But if you do it too late, you'll ejaculate, and you might get the ejaculation without the orgasm – no chills and thrills. Probably not what you want, huh?"

He smiled and agreed.

"It's easiest to do this when you're not receiving more stimulation, so tell me if you need to slow down and I'll stop touching you for a moment."

"OK."

I began caressing his chest, enjoying the fuzzy feel of the hair and the shape of his muscles. My hands moved to his flat toned belly, and past his lingam on each side to his thighs and down his legs. His lingam had softened as we talked, but as I touched him it began to stir. I caressed his inner thighs, and then moved up his belly to his chest. I lightly brushed his nipples, one with each hand. They hardened in response.

Again and again, I stroked his body, bringing awareness to each part. I lightly brushed his penis as I passed it but did not linger. I've found that the more I touch someone all over, and postpone going straight for the genitals, the more their whole body becomes involved and the easier it is for them to direct energy from the genitals to other areas.

Soon I decided that it was time to focus more on his lingam. I reached for the bottle of lubricant on the shelf behind me, and squirted some into my palm, allowing it to warm from the heat of my hand as I lightly tickled his penis with my other hand. When the lubricant was warm, I began slowly rubbing it over his lingam. After his lingam was coated, I held it gently between my two hands, pausing for a moment to allow him to feel my touch more deeply. Then both my hands began to move in swirls and curves up and down the shaft of his penis. My body danced with my hands, as I enjoyed the flow of the movement.

"Oh, slow down!" he said quickly.

Immediately I stopped, leaving my hands resting lightly just where they were.

"Breathe up to your heart," I directed him. I moved my left hand from his lingam to his heart and held it there, as he inhaled deeply and held his breath.

"Imagine that this beautiful sex energy of yours is like light opening your heart from the inside out. Let it expand your heart."

We paused motionless as he held his breath. I noticed that he was tightening his buttocks as he held his breath.

"Relax your butt. Relax your legs." I stroked them briefly to bring his attention there. "If you stay relaxed, the energy doesn't have to try to go through tight muscles. It can fill up your whole body more easily."

As he exhaled, I moved my hand back to his penis and began caressing it again. Once more his arousal built, and he asked me to stop.

"Bring it up to your heart again. Let this powerful force awaken all the love that you are capable of. Feel that love."

Inspiration struck me. "Imagine that you are holding someone in your heart. It could be a partner, a friend, or even someone you're not getting along with. Do you have someone in mind?"

He nodded, still with his eyes closed.

"Hold them there, right in the middle of all that beautiful love you have. Visualize them surrounded by your love."

A small smile crossed his face as he held his breath. A moment later, he exhaled.

"Next time when you get close, move the energy up to your third eye, right here on the center of your forehead." I touched his forehead lightly with one finger. "It's the center of visualization. You can use this powerful life force of yours to empower a goal. Right now, come up with a visual image that will represent something you'd like to have in your life. Ready?"

He nodded, and I began stimulating him again. He began to move his pelvis in pleasure.

"Slow down again," he said.

"Breathe up to the third eye. Hold it there. See your image. Feel the feelings that you'll have when this is true."

He held his breath for as long as he could. As he exhaled, I realized that I needed to tell him to include a couple of the basic laws of magic. "Often we can't even imagine the miracles that await us, so if we get too attached to the concrete image then we may limit the possibilities. Also, whatever you send out comes back to you, so it serves you to send out only good.

"So, say to yourself, 'This or something even better. And for the highest good of all concerned.'"

In a moment, I started pleasuring him. I stroked his lingam with my left hand while tickling his balls with my right fingertips. I felt his scrotum tighten and form ridges under my fingers. His balls were close to his body, and I knew he was very close to ejaculation.

"This time, I want you to just let it go. Don't try to make it happen, just allow it to happen. Try to stay as relaxed as you can so ripples can move through your whole body."

I slightly speeded up the movements of my hand on his lingam and kept a steady rhythm. Soon he began to climax. His body arched away from the table, and he moaned loudly as his cock spasmed. His head tossed from side to side. On and on it went, as he sank deeply into pleasure.

Gradually, his body quieted. He lay there, still twitching occasionally. I continued to hold his lingam softly.

"Wow! I've never experienced anything like that. That was amazing," he said, slightly dazed.

"That's what happens when you delay that many times. You're able to build to much higher levels of pleasure," I replied. "And do you see how the sexual energy can be used? It's a powerful force, and you can harness it."

"Yes, I'm beginning to see that. Thank you."

I gently disengaged from him, and went to wash my hands. I soaked a washcloth in hot water, and came back to sponge him off with reverence. I felt delighted that he had been so open to my teachings.

"Next time perhaps we'll explore the crown chakra," I told him. "Amazing things happen with the crown."

"I look forward to it."

He quietly dressed, and we said goodbye.

Shaft of Light
2004 (age 50)

"I did a phone session with Peter recently," Jeffrey told me. Peter was my partner, a remarkable man who does sexual healing work. I had recommended that Jeffrey work with him to understand more about being a man. Now Jeffrey was visiting me for another round of sessions. "He talked with me about how a man holds space for a woman. I'd like to try that with you."

I gazed at his pale round face and body, thinking how far he had come since I first met him thirteen years before. A friend who was a psychotherapist had referred him. He was her client and she had diagnosed him with Borderline Personality Disorder. He had multiple personalities. The two that I knew were Jeffrey, the adult, and Rusty, the child. They were very distinct personalities. I could usually tell by the tone of voice which one was there. Rusty's was child-like and innocent, while Jeffrey's was very depressed and wooden. When he shifted from one personality to another, his body often trembled and shook for a few moments until the other personality emerged.

His mother, who was very uncomfortable with sexuality, had abused him as a child. When he got erections in the bath, she would scrub his penis so harshly that it hurt. She also had hit his penis with a ruler. He told me one story about how she threw him down a flight of stairs when he angered her. When he was three she shut him out into the Montana winter with no coat because he had a tantrum, to teach him not to be angry.

I had learned all this gradually. It took years to build trust with him, and we spent many sessions with me holding him like a baby, so that he could learn that he was safe. I often just cupped his genitals in my hand with no stimulating touch. He said it felt "cozy."

Even as I had helped his growth, he had inspired it in me. His needs had required me to stretch into ways of working with clients that I had never done before. During one session, after about five or six years of working together, he told me about being scared of yonis *(vaginas)*. His mother had told him that there were teeth in them, and that they would bite off his vajra (his name for his penis). I had never been undressed or allowed any intimate touch with a client, but it seemed important to his healing process that I let him feel inside my yoni to see that there were no teeth.

I gave him a latex glove, and he eased it over his large hand. I took off my underwear, lifted my dress, and opened my vagina for him.

"It's so beautiful," Rusty said in awe. "Are you sure I won't slime you?"

"No, you won't. There's nothing slimy about you. Go ahead, feel inside. Just go in slowly."

He hesitantly reached out and touched me.

"It's ok," I reassured him. "You won't hurt me. And you won't be hurt. There are no teeth in there."

He slid his finger inside.

"Feel around in there. See if you can find any teeth."

15

He probed a little. "No, no teeth."

"I'm going to squeezed around your finger now. Feel that? That's as much as a yoni could do to your vajra. That wouldn't hurt, would it?"

"Nooo . . . "

Today, that fragmented man was healed enough to want to be able to give rather than receive. The years of work we had done together had produced a miraculous transformation. The fear and shame that had been wrapped up with his sexuality were largely gone. His multiple personalities were completely integrated, blending into a man who was quirky, interesting, and fun to be with. He was now ready to learn what it took to be a normal person in a healthy relationship.

I asked him, "What did you have in mind for today?"

"I want to do whatever you'd like."

I thought for a moment. I was tired from nights of insomnia. I was deeply into a transformational process, going through menopause and an astrological transit called Chiron Return. It was turning me inside out. Everything I knew about myself was no longer true. My sexuality, which had been a touch-stone my whole life, was now unpredictable and erratic. With a history of years of doing sexual surrogacy work with him, I had been concerned about this session with him, wondering how it would go, if I would even be able to be sexual with him.

"That sounds wonderful," I said in relief. "How about a massage?" I knew that he enjoyed giving massage, and that he had been to massage school.

"Sounds good. Whatever you want."

Soft music played and the light grew dim as he massaged me for about an hour. Darkness fell, and the only light was from the candles upon the altar next to the massage table. I felt myself relax more and more deeply. As I let go, I began to feel the emotions that I had been pushing away. Tears welled up in my eyes.

"I can't cry now," I thought to myself. "This is his session, not mine. It wouldn't be appropriate."

He continued to massage my low back, and the tears became unavoidable. Finally, I spoke. "I'm feeling a lot of sadness coming up. It's not about you. Is it ok if I just cry?"

"Totally fine," he said. "Cry all you want. I'd be honored."

I broke into sobs, which shook my body. Crying out my pain, my confusion, my uncertainty with who I was now, I released it all. I howled and moaned, grieving the loss of who I used to be. The tears went on and on, as I accessed what seemed like a bottomless well of sorrow. Even with my lifetime of ease with emotions, I had never wept so long or so deeply.

He moved to lie on the table beside me. Holding me in his arms, he gave comfort as I continued to sob. Finally, the tears subsided.

"That was good," he murmured to me. "You released a lot."

I looked up at him through wet eyelashes and swollen eyelids, checking how he was. He seemed centered and calm, happy to be holding me.

"Are you OK?" I asked.

"I'm good," he replied. "I'm honored that you trusted me enough to do that."

I snuggled in closer. As my naked body touched his, I began to be aroused. He responded with his own arousal. We began to move together, rubbing against each other. I moaned as I felt my yoni grow open and wet.

"Would you like to be inside me?" I asked him.

"Yes, if you want it."

"I do. I want it a lot. Let's put a condom on you."

The condom in place, I moved on top of him, placing his erect penis at the opening to my vagina. Slowly I slid down over his vajra, taking him into me at my timing and desire. Eventually he filled me, and I paused in pleasure, savoring the moment.

We began moving together, rocking our hips. My arousal grew, and I felt an orgasm near; not quite there yet, but soon. Suddenly a huge shaft of golden light entered me from my root chakra and moved up my spine, creating a wave through my body. The top of my head burst open and I became the light, loosing my sense of a personal self. I was in an exquisite union with All-That-Is, floating in ecstasy.

Timeless moments passed as we hovered in stillness. Tears of joy streamed from my eyes, and fell upon his face. Eventually, I landed back into only three dimensions.

"What was that?" he asked in wonder.

I described the shaft of light to him.

"Yes, I felt it," he said. "It was astounding." I thought to myself once again what a remarkable man he was. His perceptions of energy were extraordinary.

"Thank you so much for holding such space for me," I said in gratitude. "This was an important event for me."

"Yes, well, it was good for me too. I need to learn how to hold that space for a woman. You allowed me to be a man."

As he prepared to leave, I noticed the time. We had been together five hours, and had only scheduled two.

"I'm not going to charge you for this extra time," I told him. "It was valuable to me, and I want to acknowledge you for it."

"That feels good."

After he left, I lay on the table, reflecting upon how much the universe provides. All the care that I had poured into this man over the years had just come back to me, at the time that I needed it the most.

2 - Beginnings

A Mother's Gift
1972 (age 16)

I was sixteen years old, still a virgin. I was going to go for a vacation to the beach with my friends. I was due to have my period, so I asked my mother if I could use tampons. She got me some.

I went upstairs into the bathroom, nervous at the thought of putting something inside me. I was so tense that my muscles tightened. I couldn't get the tampon in. It hurt to try.

I was determined. After about half an hour, I finally succeeded. I emerged from the bathroom, white-faced.

My mother gazed at me quietly for a long moment, studying my face and formulating her words. Gently she said, "A man's body is not as hard as a tampon."

What a gift she gave me. She is a woman who loves sex, and she wanted to make sure that I did too. Her words reassured me that sex wouldn't hurt like putting in the tampon had. Her comfort with sexuality allowed me to enter a lifetime as a sexual priestess with less wounding than many others have. I chose her well.

A Father's Spanking
1962 (age 8)

I knelt facing the sofa, bent over it so my butt was vulnerable. My sister and brothers were beside me, also bent over the sofa. We had been for a long Sunday afternoon drive, and we were "bad" in the car. Daddy was going to spank us. I tried to put my hands over my butt, but he made me put them over my head. He stood over us, waiting, prolonging the anticipation of the pain. The suspense was dreadful. I waited for the pain to start.

My parents were young when they married. My father was twenty-two and my mother was twenty when they had me, the first child. They were almost children themselves, probably ill-equipped to deal with the pressures of four children in the space of four and an half years. With no resources for how to heal their own wounding, they did the best they could, as their parents did before them. A lineage of unconsciousness and abuse stretched through the past.

In retrospect, this event seems to be an attempt for my father to use us, his children, as a way to work out issues of feeling powerless. He was an interesting combination – shy in the world and angry at home. The pain in him was loud, thrashing around and hurting others in the process.

I sexualized this event as a way to deal with it, not an uncommon response. In later years, the same awful feeling of powerlessness and impending punishment was highly stimulating to me, and I explored it deeply.

Slaves
1966 (age 12)

"Oh, boy! No school again! Ya'll can spend the night," I said to Mira and Janice. Snow had forced the closure of school for days now, and my younger sister, Elise, and I had been inseparable with these two neighbor girls. Night after night, we had alternated between their house and ours. Tonight it was our turn again.

At eleven years old, Elise was just a year and a half younger than me, and Mira and Janice were the same ages we were. We were in that transition time, children with the stirrings of mysterious forces in our slender bodies.

Night came, and we all bedded down in the large bedroom that Elise and I shared. My mother said good night and made us turn the light out. But we were far from sleepy, wired with the excitement of being out of the usual routine.

"Let's play 'Slaves'", I whispered into the darkness. A chorus of assents was whispered back. This was a familiar game. One person became the slave, and the others got to tell them what to do. The slave had to do whatever they were told.

"Who's the first slave?" I asked, hoping that it would be me. It didn't seem right that I wanted to be a slave. It was obvious that anyone with any sense would want to be the master.

"Not me!"

"Me neither."

"How about you?"

I smiled in the dark. "Oh, ok, I'll be first. What do I have to do?"

There was a pause as the other girls thought. I felt the excitement build in me as I waited to hear what I had to do. There was a curious pleasant feeling in my . . . well, down there. I didn't have a word for it.

"Take off your clothes and stand in front of the window."

A thrill went through me. If I did that, someone driving by on the road outside might be able to see me! I didn't consider that since the room was dark, no one would be able to see in.

I stood up and removed my pink pajamas. Naked, I walked over to the window. I could see the shapes of the other girls and hear their giggles. "I hope Mama doesn't come in and tell us to be quiet," I thought to myself. "We'd really get into trouble if I'm nekkid."

My mind whirled with the lure of the forbidden. Nudity was a big taboo in our household. Knowing that I was breaking the rules added to the excitement I felt.

"How long do I have to stand here?" I asked, enjoying being subject to their whims.

"Till we tell you to stop," Mira said.

I was deeply into surrender. A profound sense of peace settled into me from being out of control. On top of the peace was arousal, nervousness at the prospect of being caught by Mama, stimulation at being naked and an edgy fear that I might be seen from the road. It was a heady mix.

Minutes passed as I sank into the moment. Finally the other girls grew bored.

"OK, you can get dressed now," Mira said.

Blinking, I came out of my semi-trance, thankful that the darkness hid my face. I shook off the feelings as I got dressed in my pajamas again.

"Whose turn is it now?"

There is a channeled entity called "Michael" who teaches a very complex system of how our souls move through lifetime after lifetime. According to "him", we choose one of seven goals each lifetime, to explore that particular facet of experience. Around my fiftieth birthday, a Michael channel told me that I have a lifetime goal of submission. I began my explorations of submission at an early age, and they continue to deepen to this day. At first, sexuality was the arena in which I played, but later in life, my form became about surrendering to the will of Spirit. "Thy will, not my will, be done."

Bondage
1995 (age 41)

"Lie down on the bed and put your arms out," Peter said in a no-nonsense voice. He tied my wrists to each side of the bed. I was naked.

My beloved and I were visiting our favorite clothing-optional hot spring resort. Forty-one years old, I was enjoying the passion of this relationship that was only two years old. Being there, watching all the naked bodies in the pools always awakened our erotic imaginations. We had decided to go back to our room for an afternoon nap.

He stood there for a moment, looking down at me with loving clear green eyes. I admired his slender muscular body and his blonde hair. He walked out of our room, leaving the door open. Our room was somewhat set back from the main walkway, but a stairway went right past our door. If someone walked by they could have seen into our room, seen me tied to the bed, squirming in arousal. They could have walked in and done whatever they wanted with me. Mmmm . . .

I watched the stairway, wondering what he was doing, when he would come back, feeling very turned on by the whole situation, my exposure, my vulnerability.

Finally he returned. He walked in and closed the door. He dropped a light pillow over my eyes so that I couldn't see.

There was silence, waiting. The tension grew. What was next? What was he going to do?

I felt a mouth on my left nipple. Soft, engulfing all of it. Sucking it up into his mouth. Mmmm, it felt good.

He stopped again. I felt no touch. There was no sound, no movement except mine. My legs were apart, open, inviting him in.

I felt the pillow being pushed slightly aside, to uncover my ear. Peter spoke softly into my ear.

"I love you so much," he said. "I want to pleasure you as much as you can receive."

My heart thrilled to hear his words. He stroked my belly, my breasts, my chest, my thighs, touching lightly and gently, just barely brushing the tips of my pubic hair. I felt so loved and cared for.

I felt a mouth on my labia. As he licked me my arousal heightened. He stopped for a moment, and then his wet fingers entered me. He began to lick again, focusing on my clit. His fingers stroked my sacred spot *(G spot)*. Waves of energy moved out from my sacred spot as I sighed in pleasure.

He played me like an instrument, sensing when I was about to come, backing off, to build my energy higher and higher without letting me come. He alternated between his tongue on my clit and his fingers on my sacred spot. My breathing came faster and faster, and each exhale was accompanied by a cry.

He kissed down my neck, licking and biting. Kissing my nipples. Pinching them. Rolling them in his fingers, pulling them up.

27

Oh, this man was such a fantastic lover. I wanted him so much. I wanted to fuck him. My cunt was aching for him.

He licked me again, burying his face in my pussy. I loved the feel of my labia around his mouth. I began to come, a tremendous rush of energy that overtook me. Toning at the top of my voice, my sounds coming from deep in my belly, from my pussy. It went on and on, huge rushes, like a stormy ocean crashing on the beach. I rode the waves of ecstasy.

As my orgasm subsided, he stopped licking me. There was a momentary pause, then I felt his cock at the entrance to my pussy. There was no resistance. I was wide open and ready for him. He slid his cock into me, easily, all the way in.

I felt his chest against mine and his hard cock inside me. So big, the perfect size. It touched me in just the right places, just the right way. He pushed in hard, staying still. Pleasure radiated out from his cock through my body. I was coming without moving externally, floating on the ripples of pleasure.

He began to move then, to fuck me. I was so open that he could easily plunge all the way in. He moved fast, pulling almost out and then driving deep inside again. With each thrust I felt full, taken, *his.*

Still with my eyes covered, I remembered a man I had seen in the pools that day. Beautiful body, black skin that had that special shine, muscular, and one of the longest cocks I have ever seen. I imagined that it was him who was fucking me; that he had walked into the room while Peter was gone, and that long thick cock was fucking me hard.

I kept coming and coming. My cries of pleasure were loud and deep. My breathing was fast. Sometimes I moved under him, fucking him. Sometimes I stayed still, letting him fuck me. The passion was wild.

Peter moved my legs up with his arms, holding them high, opening my pussy even further, plunging into me. I had never been that open. My legs were wide apart. My pussy felt bottomless. I was coming and coming and coming and coming. Waves of pleasure moved me, up my spine, out my head, down my legs. I was electricity running out in all directions from my center, my core, my sex.

My energy began to slow. Peter told me to relax, just to receive, soft belly, no tension. He licked me again. I was liquid, surrendered. There was no effort. I floated on sensation. The energy was quieter, softer.

Peter lifted the pillow enough to uncover my mouth, and slid his cock into it. I began to lick him, but he only stayed a moment.

I heard him stroking himself above me, rapid movements, faster and faster. He was breathing hard and fast. I listened to the little squishy noises as his hand moved over his cock. He began to moan.

"Stroke that hard cock," I said. "Give it to me. Let me have it. Come all over me."

His tempo quickened. He cried out, and the first warm thick drops hit my left breast. He kept coming, again and again splashing my belly, my chest, my breasts. I was covered with warm thick cream.

He moved the pillow from my eyes, and we looked at each other in wonder. He untied my wrists. I reached up and pulled him to me.

"Lie on me, let's slide in the come," I said. He lay on top of me, slipping in the slickness of his semen.

He dried us off gently. We were moving in slow motion. The warm glow of well-being washed over us both. His face was soft, wrinkles smoothed out. His eyes had depth and serenity.

The glow lasted as we packed up our things to drive back home.

On Your Knees
2004 (age 50)

"On your knees," my lover Jay said.

I looked at him, considering. Fifty years old, I was independent, no longer instantly available for whatever a man said. We were freshly out of the shower. His burgundy robe offset his dark skin and hair, and his hazel eyes twinkled at me. "This might be fun," I thought to myself. I sank to my knees in front of him. He opened his robe. His cock was beginning to stiffen. I took my time, looking at it, brushing it with the back of my hand. It got harder as I did.

I began to brush my cheek against his thigh, smelling his faint male smell. I lightly brushed my lips against his balls. I was teasing my mouth as much as I was teasing him, taking him as I desired.

I moved my cheek against his penis, feeling the smooth skin stretched over his hardness. It delighted my cheek. My lips began to part, wanting him inside my mouth. I put my lips around him, sliding him into my mouth only about an inch, feeling the spongy tip of his cock and tasting its salty slickness. I took him in deeper, filling my mouth, my passion rising as I engulfed him. He moaned.

As I continued to suck him, I became aware of the energy funneling through his cock. It spiraled from somewhere else, another dimension, as if his lingam was the spigot for this flow. It entered my throat, and moved upward and out my crown, still spiraling as it moved through me. I felt myself merge with the energy and my personal self dissolved. There was no "I", only a beautiful experience of light. My body opened from the inside out to unite with All-That-Is.

3 - First Loves

Male Love
1974 (age 20)

Mark and I lazed in his big claw-foot bathtub. He sat behind me, and I leaned into his chest. We were 20, and had been dating for about three months. I liked him, but I wasn't in love with him.

"Hey, Mark! You busy?" a man's voice came from next door.

Mark lived in a run-down Victorian house near the urban university we both attended. It had been converted to studio apartments. His was on the second floor, and the bathroom window looked out to the busy street. The voice was coming from the second floor apartment next door.

Mark got out of the tub. Water dripped down his long lean body, shining on his dark skin. He went to the window and leaned out.

"Hey, man. We're taking a bath. Want to come over in about half an hour?"

"Sure. I'll be over."

Mark returned to the tub and eased himself in behind me again.

"That was my neighbor Dave. He'll be over soon."

"OK," I replied, settling into his chest again. "That's the one you told me about who's bisexual, right?"

"Yeah, that's the one," he confirmed.

"Ever think about being sexual with him?" I murmured, rubbing my cheek against him. His cock stirred a little against my back, answering me before his words did.

"I don't know . . . maybe . . ."

"You ever been with a man before?" I asked.

"No, but I've been wondering about it," he admitted.

I turned and smiled at him, then drew him closer for a kiss. Heat began to rise between us.

"Dave'll be here soon." I broke the kiss. "We should calm down."

"OK," he said reluctantly. I turned back away from him, and our bodies relaxed.

We soaked for a while longer until the water began to get cold, and then washed each other tenderly. I enjoyed the smooth slippery feel of the soap over his skin. We rinsed and got out of the tub, drying ourselves off.

"My skin feels so soft," I said. "I don't feel like getting dressed again."

"Let's not."

"But Dave is coming."

"It'll be ok."

This was a new concept. I had never met Dave, and never been naked with anyone but a lover, and not all that many lovers, at that. I felt excited at the prospect of being daring.

"All right, let's not get dressed."

We went into the other room and lounged upon his bed. Soon Dave knocked on the door. Mark went to open it.

"We didn't feel like getting dressed. Is that ok?"

Dave looked a little shocked, but quickly recovered. "Sure, it's fine."

He walked inside to the lumpy green sofa. "I think I'll join you."

I watched as he began taking his clothes off. He was shorter than Mark, and more muscular. I appreciated the curves of his shoulders and chest as he removed his shirt. The jeans were next. Oh! No underwear! I liked that. His buttocks were round and firm, and his skin was pale and freckled.

As he turned around to sit down, I sneaked a peek at his cock. It was surrounded by beautiful blonde hair, which matched the hair on his head.

"Very nice!" I thought to myself.

I was quiet as they chatted about a class they shared. I didn't quite know how to be in this situation. I felt attracted to both of them, but I wasn't sure what either of them was expecting. What did they want? What did I want?

I decided to be daring. "Let's all get in bed together."

They looked at me for an instant, surprised at my suggestion. Then they exchanged glances, as if searching for something. Permission from the other, maybe? I wasn't sure.

After a moment, Mark got up. He reached his hand out to me and pulled me up. I extended my hand to Dave, encouraging him up as well. We all walked over to Mark's bed and he pulled back the covers.

"I want to be in the middle," I said, sliding across the white sheets. Dave joined me on my right, and Mark crawled over me to my left. We snuggled in together, my arms around each of their necks. They put their arms across my belly and chest.

The novelty of being in bed with two men had me instantly excited. At the same time, it felt completely natural and easy.

I turned to Mark and kissed him deeply. Dave pressed against my back as my body moved in response to Mark's kiss. I moaned as Dave nibbled my neck.

Finishing my kiss with Mark, I turned to Dave, with Mark's arms still around me and his body close to mine. I looked into Dave's green eyes for a moment, and saw goodness looking back. He began to kiss me, gently at first, and then with more passion. I met his passion with my own. My body heated and my breathing quickened.

"Now you two should kiss," I said.

There was another long moment as they looked at each other. They each lifted up on an elbow. Dave reached across me to the back of Mark's head, and drew him close. I watched as their lips met right above my face. I was immersed in the fascination of seeing two men kissing.

As they continued their kiss, I took in the contrast between them. Dave's fair skin intensified Mark's darkness as their cheeks were so close together. Their shining wet tongues met as their lips parted. They were beautiful in their passion.

They turned their heads towards me, and we joined in a three-way kiss. I began to moan as our tongues played with each other. I pulled them close to me, wriggling in arousal. Their hands roamed across my body, touching my belly, my breasts, my pubic hair. One of their hands, I wasn't sure whose, slid onto the surface of my hot, wet pussy. I opened my legs more to allow him in, and I moved my arms so I could take their erect cocks in each hand. I rubbed their penises on my hips, feeling the wet trail of fluid that they left behind.

Mark began to kiss my breasts as I kissed Dave's mouth. He slowly moved down my chest, my belly, my hips, to my yoni. I turned slightly to my side, spreading my legs further apart for Mark, as I began to lick Dave's nipples. They stiffened in response, and he gasped in pleasure. As Mark began to move his tongue all around my pussy, it swelled and got hotter. I continued my pathway down Dave's body, licking and nibbling his firm flat belly, and finally reaching my destination – that beautiful golden nest of pubic hair. I nuzzled my face into the curls, inhaling his scent deeply. His pelvis moved and his erect cock called to me. I took it into my mouth, tasting the saltiness at the tip, as Mark's tongue pulled me more and more deeply into pleasure.

"Let's shift around here so I can suck you," Dave said to Mark.

We adjusted our positions so that we were lying in a triangle, mouths to genitals. As Dave engulfed Mark's penis with his mouth, I slid my mouth back down onto Dave's cock and Mark resumed his delicious attention to my pussy. I felt us

37

building together, as energy flew around the triangle. My body began to ripple in orgasm. I lost Dave's penis from my mouth as I screamed in passion.

"I want to fuck you both," I said with a profound desire in my body. "How about you in my ass, Mark, and Dave in my pussy?"

They agreed with delight. Mark lay down on his back, and I stretched my body out on top of him with my back to him. Dave sat on his knees between both our legs, and moistened Mark's cock with his saliva. He guided it into my anus. I was so open and excited that it went in easily.

"Now you, Dave," I said in a voice deepened with desire.

He leaned forward with his hands on either side of my shoulders, and positioned his penis so that he slid effortlessly into my slippery vagina. I had never felt so full.

Dave's mouth met mine as we all began to move together. My arms went around him, and I felt Mark's arms encircle us both. The three of us rocked in one rhythm, with passion building rapidly. Dave moved his mouth from mine to Mark's, and I felt the electricity of their kiss beside my ear. My moans joined theirs as the fire escalated. We exploded into orgasm together, shouting as waves of delight ran through us.

As the passion ebbed, we lay there together with our arms around each other, quivering with aftershocks. I felt close and connected to them, and deeply honored to be present at Mark's awakening into loving a man.

The Pick-Up
1976 (age 22)

It was a warm spring Saturday night in Virginia, and I was feeling the tides of desire surging. I was 22, fully caught up in the sexual exploration of the times, the wild seventies. At home with Wade, my first husband, I felt a longing for some excitement. We had settled into the same evening we always had, smoking pot and watching television. The heaviness of boredom hung over me. He had encouraged my experiments before, so I imagined that he would again.

"I'm going to go out and pick up somebody," I said to him, beginning to dress in a blue plaid shirt. I left a few buttons open and I wore no bra.

He looked surprised. "What are you going to do?"

"I'm going to find somebody and have sex with him," I answered, pulling on my short jean skirt.

"Are you going to bring him back here?" he asked warily.

"No, I'll go to his place," I answered, not wanting to displace him from his home.

"All right," he said. His wiry body was tight, and his jaw was twitching, but then, it usually was. I didn't probe any further into how he was feeling.

Our relationship was a convoluted one, sexually. He had originally encouraged me to be sexual with others. At first I

39

was surprised at the idea, and he had convinced me that he wanted it. After some resistance, I had decided to experiment with it. His reactions were not always positive, but sometimes he seemed to enjoy it. We didn't talk much about how we felt with each other.

Sliding on my sandals, I walked out the door and onto the city street, feeling adventuresome and on the prowl. I had never done anything like this before.

I strolled a couple of blocks, watching the faces of the other students as I walked by the funky little shops in this commercial neighborhood near the university that I attended. Who would it be? I felt aroused at how daring I was being.

My eyes fell upon a man I had met a week before on the block where I lived. He was tall, with long hair, expressive brown eyes, and full sensual lips. We had held a brief conversation about numerology while our glances at each other had lingered.

"Steve! Hi!" I called out to him. He turned and smiled at me.

"Hi! What are you doing tonight?" he asked.

"Not much," I replied, moving closer to him and looking at him seductively. "Would you like to go back to your place?"

He agreed, and we turned and walked back to his apartment. It had only been about ten minutes since I had left my building. I was surprised at how quickly I had found someone, and a little disappointed that the excitement of the hunt was over. We entered his apartment, and a large fluffy white cat jumped off the windowsill and greeted us. The place was cluttered with books, plants, and a few discarded items of clothing. He obviously hadn't been expecting a guest.

I eyed him hesitantly, a mix of feelings churning through me. "Maybe I shouldn't be here. I don't even know him. Maybe I should be home with Wade instead. But I started this already. And he's pretty cute. What the hell . . .I can always go home to Wade later. He'll like to fuck me."

He reached out and pulled me into a long wet kiss. My thoughts evaporated as an instant surge of heat overtook me. I began panting as my whole body strained up towards him. He pulled me closer, and we pressed the full length of our bodies together. I felt his penis stiffen and push into my belly.

I broke the kiss, and looked up at him intently. He took my hand and led me into his bedroom. The bed was disheveled, but I didn't care. We fell upon it, our mouths meeting hungrily again. Still kissing me, he pulled my blouse from my skirt, and reached underneath, cupping my breast in his hand. He tweaked the nipple, and I moaned. Already I felt warmth and wetness in my pussy, and I parted my legs. He put one of his legs in between mine and pressed up against my clitoris. I began to move against his thigh. My arms pulled him tight as my body reached up to him.

His hand left my blouse and moved under my skirt, finding my soaked panties. He reached inside them, and slid his finger easily along my swollen slit. I moaned again. Oh, it felt good!

I thrust in rhythm with his hand. Soon an orgasm stiffened my legs as I pulsed around his finger, and I cried out in pleasure.

As my orgasm subsided, I wanted more. We fumbled with clothing, and quickly were naked. Parting my legs, I drew him close, pulling against his curvy buttocks as he pressed deeply into me. I was wet and open, and he filled my emptiness.

We were locked in the ancient dance that was so new in this moment. His cock slid back and forth inside me as we kissed passionately and deeply. Passion built, and another orgasm overtook me. I let out a wordless yell as it went on and on.

My body became limp and exhausted, but he was not finished. He turned me over, grabbing my hips and lifting my butt up so that he could enter me again. My face pressed into the pillow, and I sagged from his hands. But as he plunged into me over and over, my own excitement awoke. I began meeting his thrusts with my own, arching my back so that I was open even wider for him. Faster and faster we moved, building to an intensity that sent us both over the edge. Together we came, in an explosion of delight.

We collapsed onto the bed. I was still face down and he was on top of me. Soft pillows surrounded my face and it was a little hard to breathe. We lay there together until his weight became too much, and then I squirmed out from under him.

"That was really great," I murmured to him. Sighing, I rubbed my eyes. They felt a little itchy.

We rested for a while, not talking. My sinuses were starting to feel irritated, and my nose began to run. I sneezed.

"I'm not feeling so great," I said. "I feel like I'm allergic to something. Is there cat hair on the pillow?"

"Probably," he said. "I'm sorry."

"That's OK. I should go home now." I slid out of bed and picked up my clothes. He lay there as I dressed in silence. The ecstasy of the previous moment had evaporated and I felt miserable, sneezing and my eyes running.

"Well, see you around," I said, walking out the bedroom door. "I'll just let myself out."

I walked into the night, depressed and empty. My adventure had been fun in the moment, but I was already regretting it. How would Wade react? Why had I done it? My allergic eyes were streaming the tears of pain I refused to cry.

A few days later, a place on my labia began to hurt. Was it a pimple? An infected hair follicle? I let it go for a day or two, and as the pain got more and more intense, I made an appointment with my gynecologist.

"It's a new virus called herpes," he said. "You'll have it the rest of your life."

Despondent, I left his office. "I can't bear this. I can't live with this kind of pain," I thought to myself. He had neglected to tell me that the lesions would go away, and I thought that it would always hurt that much.

The pain of the herpes was a physical manifestation of the inner pain I felt about my sexuality. The atmosphere of free love that permeated the seventies contradicted the way that I was raised to believe that sex was only for your husband. I wanted to be a free spirit, both because the times were asking for it and because I had so much desire, but I was laden with generations of conditioning. I viewed contracting herpes as a fitting punishment for my sins, even though I wanted to go out and sin again! My gynecologist's response fit into this paradigm. Unsympathetic, he was like a judge pronouncing my sentence.

Young and unsure of myself, I believed that my value was in my sexuality. I found a kind of validation in my attractiveness, an affirmation that I was worth something after all. It was an area in which I felt confident and competent, unlike the rest of my life.

Bad Trip Leads to a Larger Trip
1977 (age 23)

I stood at the top of the wooden fire escape that served as the back stairs to the apartment that I shared with Wade. The old gray steps seemed to elongate and I felt dizzy as I looked down.

Our friend Matt had visited earlier, bringing some kind of white powder that he said was THC. It was the seventies, and drug experimentation was ubiquitous in my circles. We all sniffed it, and he had taken off, going to give it to some other friends. Wade and I still had other guests, and they all decided to go visit Chick, another friend. I didn't want to leave the house, but I went along reluctantly because everyone else did.

I made it down the stairs, clutching the railing tightly as my vision shifted perspective. The stairs zoomed long and short. Finally I reached the bottom, and got in the car with a pile of others. Wade drove through the crowded urban streets, filled with pedestrians and bicyclists as well as cars. Everything was moving so fast! Panic filled me as I watched a line of orange cones blocking off a lane. Would he be safe? Too much input!

By the time we got to Chick's house, about a mile away, I was overwhelmed with fear. Someone helped me into his house, and I collapsed onto his living room floor, hyperventilating. My hands drew up towards my face in tetany as the hyperventilation continued. Chaos was all around me, people talking loudly and moving seemingly at random.

Finally, Wade came over to me and took my hands. "Are you OK? Do you want to go back home?"

"Yes, I really do."

"All right, I'll take you."

We walked back out to the car, and made the short trip back. When we arrived, we walked up the stairs, and I gratefully entered our living room. I curled up in a little ball on the sofa, still under the influence of the drug, which was now creating a grinding contraction in my head, as if something was pushing upon the back of my skull.

"This is scary," I said. "I don't like this at all."

He didn't reply. He flung himself into a chair, slouching there for a moment. His face twitched in its usual tic. He jumped up again, his wiry body filled with nervous energy as he moved quickly around the apartment.

"I'm going out again. This is no fun being here."

"But I don't want to be alone! I'm scared."

"You'll be all right," he said. "I'll be back later."

The door closed behind him, and I felt abandoned. Helpless to do anything about the unpleasant effects of the drug I had taken, I was out of control. Panic threatened to return. I tried to relax, to reassure myself that I would be all right once the drug wore off.

There was a knock at the door, and Matt entered again.

"Matt! Thank god! I'm so glad to see you!" I cried. I didn't know him well, but I was glad to see anyone at that point. He had always been fun to be around, very light-hearted and playful. With his Dutch accent he was somewhat of a novelty in this southern city. His pale skin and thick glasses were a reminder of his night owl habits.

"Where's Wade?"

"He left. He said it wasn't any fun being here with me. I've been having a hard time with this drug."

"He left you?" he asked in disbelief. "You need someone here with you. I'll stay."

"Oh, thank you so much."

He sat down beside me and stroked my shoulder. I felt myself melt a little under his touch.

"Are you sure that was THC?" I asked.

"No, it might not have been. That's what the person told me who gave it to me, but I don't really know. It could have been PCP."

"I really need to start being more careful about what I take," I thought to myself. "I don't want to do this again."

We waited through the night together, talking quietly, getting to know each other. I felt safe with him, and I knew that he wouldn't leave me. The sky was getting gray by the time I began come down from the drug.

"Do you want to watch the sun rise?" I asked him.

"Sure."

I led him out to the balcony. He sat on the floor with his back to the wall, and I settled in between his legs, leaning against his chest. He wrapped his arms around me and I felt peace ease through me. This man, who hardly knew me, had done me a great service that night, more than my husband had been willing to do. My heart opened to him.

Not long after that, we became lovers. He was an innocent, with little experience with women, but he had a very loving heart. Later, he was there to help me through the divorce with Wade, holding me as I cried and then making me laugh. I was grateful for his companionship and love.

After a few months, he got a job in Washington, DC. He asked me to move there with him. I was stunned at the possibility. I had never considered that I might leave my hometown, so close to my family and all that I knew. I debated for a short while, and then said yes. The horizons of my life widened enormously.

Kicking the Habit
1977 (age 23)

Wham! I went from sleep to seeing stars. Jolted awake, adrenaline surged through me, and I began to try for protection by covering myself with my arms. He was over me, his eyes crazed. Blows came from both sides.

"I want you to hurt as much as you hurt me," Wade said with hate on his face. He continued to strike me. I kicked up at him, trying to get him off.

"Wade, stop!" I cried. He acted as if he didn't hear me. "Wade!"

His slaps rained over me. Frantic, I struggled to get away, but he was stronger and heavier. I was trapped. Eventually, he stopped hitting me and flung himself onto his back beside me.

Shaken and stunned, I began to cry. Part of me was horrified at what had just happened, and part of me felt that I deserved it. I had told him earlier that evening about a casual sexual encounter that I had that same day. He had reacted with anger and pain. We had argued well into the night until finally I had said that I needed to sleep. After dozing for a while, this was how I had awakened.

"Take me to him!" he demanded.

"I can't do that!" I thought to myself. "I can't involve Nick. It's the middle of the night. I barely know him. But Wade is crazy. I'm afraid of him. Maybe I could just stay there with Nick once we get there. I could tell him that Wade just beat me, and maybe he would help me."

"OK, I'll take you there," I acquiesced.

In silence, we dressed and walked out to the car. I sat as far from him as possible. We drove through the dark streets to Nick's apartment, and walked up the stairs to his door. Wade banged on the door, and a few moments later, a sleepy-eyed Nick opened it. In shock, he looked from my battered face to Wade's angry one.

"I want you to know that you fucked my woman," Wade said confrontationally. "If you ever go near her again, you'll be sorry."

"OK, man, no problem," he said, raising his hands in front of him in peace and taking a step backwards.

"Now's the time," I thought to myself urgently. "I need to say something now to get his help." I remained silent, not sure if it was right to involve him any more than he already was.

"Come on!" Wade grabbed my arm and pulled me around to walk away. Numb, I went with him. My chance had passed.

Back at home, we undressed for bed in silence. Nervous, I slept as far away from him as possible.

The next morning, I looked in the bathroom mirror. My lip was swollen, and I had slight bruises around my eye. Tears streamed down as I contemplated the damage of the night, both to my face and to our relationship.

I walked back into the bedroom where he was. "If you ever hit me again, I'm leaving."

He just stared at me stonily.

The doorbell rang, and I went to answer it. My sister was dropping in unexpectedly. I invited her in reluctantly, not wanting to tell her what had happened. The three of us sat uneasily in the living room. Wade emanated cold anger, and I sat there in a daze as she tried to make conversation.

"Can she see what happened to my face?" Guilt poured through me. I felt like a slut. If she knew the situation she would disapprove of me.

After a short time, she took her leave without ever saying anything about what was going on with me. Perhaps she was adhering to our family's unwritten rule: don't bring up anything controversial. Keep to the surface, it's safer. I got ready for work, and left the house with a sense of escape.

Things continued to deteriorate between Wade and myself over the next three weeks. One day, we stood in the dining room, shouting at each other.

"If you don't watch it, I'll hit you!" he threatened me.

"Ooooh, big tough man! I'm so scared!" I taunted him.

He reached out and lightly slapped my face. It was almost a token jab, not really meant to do damage like the time before.

"That's it! I'm leaving!" I announced, with a sense of relief that this disaster of a relationship was over. I realized that I had pushed him to hit me again so that I would have an excuse to leave.

I packed up a few of my things, and went to stay at a friend's house. Within a week, I had found a new place to live, and had moved my things there. Once that was done, I never went back.

When I left him, it was a step from darkness into the light. As I began living with the woman friend who took me in, I began to find myself again, my likes and desires. I cooked a dinner of chicken livers and corn – food that he hated – and celebrated my independence.

After a few weeks, I stayed home from work one day with a cold. I had no cigarettes all day, which was unusual because I had smoked heavily since I had met Wade. It was a lovely spring afternoon, and as I started feeling better I walked down to the corner store to buy a pack. Back home, I lit one up, and immediately felt worse. The thought came to me, "I don't have to kill myself anymore. I'm free of him."

I stopped smoking that day, and never did again.

Newly a Virgin
1978 (age 24)

"Let's pretend I'm a virgin and you're going to initiate me," I said to Travis, my future second husband. We had been lovers for less than a year, enjoying affection and passion in many expressions.

His heart-shaped face lit up, and his brown eyes sparkled. "Sounds like fun."

My mind drifted back to the real first time with my boyfriend Mike when I was sixteen years old – both of us virgins, inexperienced, fumbling, rushed. When it was over, all too soon, I asked him, "Did we do it?"

Now, in my early twenties, I knew that it would be different with Travis. He was a considerate and skilled lover, and enjoyed my pleasure as much as his own.

He took my hand and led me to the bed. Sinking into my role, I perched there hesitantly. He sat beside me, placing a hand on my cheek as he looked into my eyes with love.

"I want this first time to be really special for you," he said tenderly. "I want you to really enjoy it. You tell me if there's anything you want, or if something doesn't feel right. OK?"

"OK," I replied, still nervous, thinking to myself. "Will it hurt? Will I enjoy it? I love him so. I want to do this."

He pulled me closer and began to lightly kiss my face. His lips brushed my forehead, my eyelids, as he held my head with both his hands. His beard grazed my cheek, and I caught my breath. My lips parted, and he moved closer to gently touch them with his own. Our breath mingled.

I reached my lips up to him and he met them, still with my face between his hands. He moved his head so that his dry lips rubbed mine. He slid his wet tongue out of his mouth and lightly tickled the inside of my upper lip. A wave of desire rushed through me, and my whole body stretched to be closer to him.

"Gently, my dear, let's take our time," he murmured softly. "There's never going to be another first time. Let's make it last."

I took a deep breath. All fear had left me, and I was eager and excited to be with him totally – to become a woman.

I lay back on the white bedspread and reached my arms out to him. He came into them, lying close to my right side. He began to kiss me again. This time, the kisses were deeper. His tongue met mine and swirled around it. I wrapped my arms around him and held him tight.

At last, the kiss ended. He raised his head and looked into my eyes. "I love you," he said, putting his heart into his words.

"I love you too," I answered, filled to overflowing with the truth of it.

He began to kiss the place where my jaw met my neck, then traveled down the line of muscle to the little hollow above my collarbone. From there, he nuzzled my chest, just above my breast.

"May I unbutton your blouse?" he asked.

"Yes," I replied with a throaty voice.

He unbuttoned the first button of my pink blouse and kissed the part of my chest that became exposed. Another button, and the upper part of my breast appeared. Cupping it through my blouse with one hand, he traced the curve with his lips.

"Mmmm . . . beautiful. You are so lovely," he said to me.

I smiled at him as he unbuttoned the rest of my blouse and parted it. Bra-less, my rosy nipples stood up slightly. He leaned over and, holding both breasts on either side of his head, kissed my heart and rubbed his face on my breasts. His beard tickled me softly. A quiet purr came from me.

Still holding my breasts, he moved to my left nipple and just touched it with the tip of his tongue. I gasped.

"You like that?" he asked, looking up at me.

"Oh, yes," I said eagerly. "Do it some more!"

He returned to the same nipple and licked it with his soft tongue. Still looking at me, he kissed and sucked on it until I began to squirm.

"You're a hot little thing to be a virgin," he smiled at me.

"Well, you're making me that way," I smiled back. "It's really good."

He moved to my other nipple, sucking on it more firmly and sending currents of electricity straight to my pelvis. My lips swelled open.

His tongue traveled from my breast to a spot just below my belly button. He stopped there and gently bit a roll of skin.

"I love your round woman's belly," he said. "It's so sexy."

"He likes it?" I wondered to myself. "I thought it was supposed to be flat like all the models. Hmmm . . . maybe he's telling the truth. He sure seems to like it. Wow."

He unzipped my jeans. His tongue traced a line from my belly button to the top of my lavender cotton bikini panties and slipped slightly underneath the elastic waistband. I could feel him licking the top of my pubic hair. My pussy was wet and open.

He pulled my jeans and underwear down all in one swoop, throwing them onto the floor. He stood and quickly removed his own T-shirt and jeans. I looked at his compact muscular body and his erect cock that was twitching slightly. A thrill went through me, and I lay there before him, my legs spread apart, moving in arousal. The scent of my pussy filled the air. He stood on his knees in between my legs, looking down at me with desire.

"I'm going to lick you for a very long time," he said. "I'm going to lick you until you really want to fuck me."

His words sent a rush of warmth through my body and I moved before him. He settled in between my legs, looking up at me with love. He inhaled my scent, and closed his eyes for a moment, savoring it.

Then he lightly brushed his lips across my pubic hair, kissing me softly on my belly and thighs. As he did, it was as if my vagina became an open honeysuckle blossom. I longed for his touch.

My labia parted and he placed a soft warm kiss right in the center of them, just below my clitoris. Nuzzling me, he sank deeper into my softness. His tongue snaked out and explored my folds.

"Mmmmm . . ." he hummed. "You taste good."

I moaned in reply, and opened my legs a little wider. His hands grabbed my hips firmly and lifted me up slightly, immersing his face in me like a ripe persimmon. The tip of his tongue touched my clitoris and found it hard. He put his lips around it and sucked slightly, as his tongue tickled it. Soon, I was building towards an orgasm, but he backed off, licking lower down into my opening. Again and again he built me up and let me down, until finally I dissolved into a huge rush of fire. The orgasm plowed through me, leaving me limp and quivering.

He gathered me into his arms, lying on top of me, kissing me deeply. I smelled the musk of my pussy on his beard. He moved so that the tip of his cock was poised right at the opening to my vagina.

"Are you ready?" he asked me gently.

"Yes," I replied, slightly hesitantly, remembering my virgin role.

"Never let a man take you before you're ready. We men can wait, and it's better for us if we do."

"I'm ready. I want you inside of me. Just go slow."

"I will," he promised. He moved so that the smooth tip of his penis caressed the length of me like a finger. Gently, gradually, he placed his cock exactly at the right angle to enter me. He let me open at my own pace, meeting any resistance with stillness and patience. Because he didn't force it, his penis slipped in easily and soon I felt the tremendous relief of being filled. My hips arched up to meet him and our mouths dissolved into a deep kiss. My legs wrapped around his knees, pulling my pelvis up tighter against him. I was open and wet as we moved together, energy mounting in each of us. In rhythm, we swayed, building, building, until an orgasm began to shriek through me. It set him off as well, and both of us merged into a huge wave of pleasure. We cried out in delight, clutching each other close.

"Wow, that was incredible," I said to him as we calmed down. I snuggled in close to him. "You were so wonderful. It was just the way it should have been."

He smiled at me. "You deserve no less than that."

Transition
May, 1982 (age 28)

"I got accepted!" I looked up at Travis from the letter from the natural health college.

"Yee ha!" he raised his fist high. "We're in!"

I thought to my self, "We? I'm the one who's going to school. Oh, well, I'll just let that go. He's going to the west coast with me."

We jumped up and down and hugged each other in celebration. The year of night school had paid off. It was time to drop my computer programmer job and pursue my dream of a career as a health professional.

September, 1982

"Fifty percent of you who are married now will not be by the time your schooling is over," the professor said on orientation day.

"That won't be me," I said to myself. "I love Travis. I'm going to stay with him."

I was wrong.

We lasted for a couple of years. As I went to school, he settled into the sameness of a full-time job. I began growing and expanding my horizons as I was exposed to new people and ideas. The communication gap widened.

One rainy winter day, we looked at each other and knew that we were at the end. We took the day off, and went out into the mountains together. The rain dripped down as we walked and talked with each other, recognizing how far apart we had grown. Sadness weighed us down.

We stopped on the trail, hugging each other, with love in our hearts even as we knew that we would part. Tears streamed down both our faces, mingling with the rain.

"The sky is crying with us," he said, holding me close.

4 - Tantra

Doing It Right
1990 (age 36)

"Come on over and I'll teach you Tantra," Paul said. He was a short round man with friendly brown eyes.

"What's Tantra?" Andrew asked.

"It's a kind of sacred sexuality," Paul explained. "It uses breathing to open up your energy. I've been taking Tantra workshops for years."

Andrew and I looked at each other. His hazel eyes showed a mix of hope and fear, and he drew me close to his long lean yogi's body. Sex was a stumbling block for us. For the five years of our relationship, we had struggled with his feelings that I abandoned him when I orgasmed. I had tried modulating my passion so that he could feel included, but what had happened instead was that the passion had died. We rarely had sex, and when we did I was not orgasmic, because I was too afraid of "leaving him" again. I was often sad and frustrated about how our sex life had withered. Perhaps this would help us.

"I'd love to," I said softly.

"Me too," Andrew agreed.

The appointed evening arrived, and Andrew and I went to Paul's house. He introduced us to his girlfriend Ellen, a beautiful young woman with a vivacious face and a curvy body. We sat in a small circle, and he showed us what to do.

"Start by moving your hips like this," he rocked his pelvis. We followed his lead.

"Breathe in when you arch your back and out when your pelvis thrusts forward. Yes, that's it."

"Now, let that motion travel up your spine." His spine began to undulate with the movement of his hips. We followed suit.

"Let the motion move all the way up your neck so that your head moves. That's right," he encouraged. "Let your jaw relax."

"Wow! There's a lot of stuff to remember here!" I thought to myself.

"Let some sounds come out," Paul coached. "Sound helps the energy to move."

I opened my mouth and the next time I exhaled, a small sound came through. I continued to rock my pelvis, breathing in time to the rocking, feeling my spine undulating with the movements. Energy was starting to build. I felt like I was going to have an orgasm. I looked at my companions. None of them seemed to be in the same place I was. Perhaps I was doing it wrong? This didn't seem appropriate. I suppressed my energy and concentrated on moving correctly.

The energy built more, and I continued to suppress it, until suddenly I could hold it back no more. An orgasm overtook me, and I felt myself soar in ecstasy for several long moments. When I came back, they were all staring at me.

"Boy!" Paul exclaimed. "You really got it!"

"I did?" I faltered. "That was ok?"

"Yes, more than ok. That's what's supposed to happen! You're a natural!"

"Oh." I digested this information. "I thought I was doing it wrong."

"No, it was really right."

Andrew looked at me enviously.

The Tantric Ritual
1990 (age 36)

Andrew and I dressed together for the Tantric ritual. We were in our first Tantra workshop, soon after Paul's lesson in undulation. We had been through a day of exercises in breathing and movement designed to help us open up our sexual energy. Interspersed throughout the day, our instructor had talked about how sexuality had been honored in the past, how people had come to the temple to be instructed in the arts of love. My head was full from so many new ideas, and although I had enjoyed the day, I felt a little nervous about the evening's activities. I wasn't sure what to expect.

"How do I look?" I asked Andrew. They had instructed all of us to dress as gods and goddesses. People all around us were adorning themselves with scarves and jewelry, having fun with playing dress-up.

"I think you should have one breast bare," he dared me, pulling on the scarf that I had tied around my chest.

I took a quick glance around. Other people were skimpy in their attire. "I guess that's ok," I assented. This was new ground for both of us.

"You look good." He gave me a quick hug.

I went into the bedroom and slid my diaphragm inside. I wasn't sure if we were going to be sexual in the ritual, but I wanted to be prepared.

All the participants lined up, ready to enter the temple space. A workshop assistant came by with blindfolds.

"We're asking you to wear these so that your other senses will be heightened. You'll be led into the temple and placed with your partner."

I took a last look at Andrew. He looked handsome, with his bare chest and muscular arms. He was wearing a purple scarf draped around his waist. I put the blindfold in place, and stood there quietly. Soon someone came and took my arm.

"Please come this way," she murmured. We walked down a short hallway and went into a room that felt small. I was guided to sit down upon a bench, and I felt someone sit beside me. I assumed that it was Andrew.

Someone took my foot in his hand and placed it in a basin of warm water. I relaxed as he gently washed my foot. He ended by putting my toe in his mouth and swirling his tongue around it. Waves of sensation ran through my body, and my breathing quickened. After a moment, he stopped, and repeated the process with the other foot. Judging from the sounds beside me, Andrew was receiving the same treatment.

When the foot-washing was done, my escort drew me up by my arm, and led me into the big workshop room. Exotic music was playing.

"Welcome to the temple," someone said in low tones.

I was led to a place in the room, and soon Andrew joined me. We reached out and touched each other's hands, finding some comfort in the familiar touch while everything else was so new.

I could sense the others around me, hearing the shuffles and whispers as people got settled. Gradually the room quieted.

"Welcome to the temple of love." The voice of the workshop leader came over the microphone. "Please find a way to connect with your partner."

Andrew and I moved closer into a seated hug. Following instructions, we took a deep breath together. I felt the nervousness begin to melt away as we continued to breathe with each other.

"Let your bodies undulate together." Earlier in the day, we had practiced the same undulation technique that Paul had taught us, and learned how to do it together to raise sexual energy. I moved into Andrew's lap, and we began moving together.

All around us, I could hear the arousing sounds of sighs and moans from other couples. As we continued to undulate, I felt a feather tickle my back, then across my shoulder. "Where did that come from?" I wondered, but I stayed in the erotic trance that was building in me. I assumed that the same thing was happening with Andrew.

I could sense people moving around us, weaving a dance between all the couples. Some people stroked me with furs, other with feathers. Some lifted my long hair and let it fall around my shoulders. It was a sensory overload. I gave up trying to identify who might be touching me or what might be happening, and just abandoned myself to the pleasure.

As Andrew and I became more aroused, we moved closer to each other, pulling our bodies tight together, rubbing our chests together sensually. I could feel his erect lingam pushing at me, and I easily slid onto it as I sat in his lap. We moved together, our passion building as feathers and furs delighted every part of our bodies. Soon I cried out in orgasm, and he joined me.

As we slowed, we stayed connected, holding each other close. All around us, we could hear cries of pleasure. What an amazing scene!

Soon the workshop leader invited us to take off our blindfolds. As I did, Paul was right there, hugging me. He had been one of the assistants with the feathers.

"You are both so beautiful!" he said lovingly. "It was a pleasure to serve you."

The next morning, the group sat in a circle to talk about the night before. Andrew began to share his experiences.

"This workshop has saved our marriage," he declared. "We've had so much problems with sex, and last night it was magical."

I glowed with pleasure at hearing what he said.

Alas, the opening was short-lived. Soon the old habits asserted themselves. We never did another workshop, although they were available to us. I think that somehow I knew that it would be the end of our relationship if we pursued Tantra together, and I chose to try to save the relationship. It was challenging. We argued a lot, and sex faded away.

About a year later, he woke me on our anniversary. "This has been the worst year of my life."

"Me, too," I admitted, hurt that he would greet me that way on our anniversary. "Let's stop."

A week later, I moved out, and soon I began a new life. I moved into a new place, and started going to Tantra workshops again. Soon I was assisting in them, and taking my place in the Tantra community. Life expanded in ways that I had never imagined.

Leaving My Body Behind
1991 (age 37)

I walked into the mansion where the Tantra workshop was already in progress downstairs. It was mid-day on Saturday, and they had been together since the night before. More than a year had passed since my first Tantra workshop with Andrew, and he and I had separated a few months before. I had not been in this luxurious home overlooking the water since the first workshop. Paul had invited me to be an assistant at this weekend. I had agreed, but I had not been able to get there until this time because of work. I paused for a moment in the deserted living room, feeling nervous at what I might find and wondering how I might fit in. I took a deep breath, and made my way downstairs to the workshop room.

There were about forty people sitting in a circle. Many were dressed only in sarongs. I felt awkward and overdressed in my street clothes, but I took a place in the circle. One of the workshop facilitators was leading the group in a simple song.

"I am opening, I am opening, I am opening to love."

As the song repeated, I grew calmer, beginning to feel a part of the group. I looked around the circle at the beaming faces. Most were strangers to me, but we were creating a web between us as we sang the same song. I saw Paul across the room and he smiled at me in greeting.

When the song was over, the leaders began to teach the next exercise, a breathing technique for partners. After the introduction, they asked people to find a partner to practice. I stayed on the sidelines, wanting to just observe how I should be, since I was in new territory and unsure of myself.

One of the male participants asked a beautiful blonde woman assistant named Hope to partner with him. I remembered her from my workshop. He seemed revolting to me, obese with a distorted face. He looked like someone who would slobber all over her. She smiled and agreed to be his partner. Inwardly, I gulped in dismay. Did I have to do that too?

Sitting against the wall, I scanned the room. All around me couples were sitting together, breathing and moving with each other. Most women were in their partner's lap. Under the guidance of the leaders, the room was escalating in sexual vibrations. People were moaning in pleasure.

I looked back at the grotesque man. Hope had taken off her sarong, and her breasts were bare. The man was burying his face in them, kissing and licking with fervor. I was shocked. Is this what was expected? Did I have to offer myself to any man who was there? I watched uneasily as she gave herself to him. Partly I admired her for being able to embrace him so completely. Partly I felt repulsed at the idea that I might have to do that too.

Eventually the exercise ended, and people went off into a break. Paul came over and gave me a hug.

"Good to see you," he squeezed me firmly. I relaxed a little under his touch. "How are you?"

"Good," I said, hoping that he would believe me.

I was in a new world, trying to fit in. When I had done the last workshop with Andrew, I had partnered with him for the exercises. Since we had been in relationship, it was much more comfortable to do these things. Now I was here alone, trying to belong. I felt like an imposter. Everyone else seemed so comfortable. Was there something wrong with me?

The break over, we went back inside for the next teaching. Again, the instructors asked people to pair up to practice. This time, a young man asked me to partner with him. He had short black hair and his eyes shied away from mine. Even though I didn't feel much initial connection with him, I remembered Hope and I agreed.

We sat on the floor in front of each other, guided by the voice of the instructor coming over the microphone. Soft music played in the background. Looking into each other's eyes, we began to breathe together. My discomfort eased a little as we breathed. The instructor suggested that people move so that the women were sitting in the men's laps. With a little nervousness, I complied.

As the instructor coached us to intensify our breathing to make the energy hotter, he grabbed my hips. His penis was erect and bumping into my yoni through our clothing. He thrust against me forcefully over and over. I felt myself deaden and leave my body. It was as if I was not even there. I had just left a shell sitting upon his lap with a smile frozen on its face.

Finally the exercise was over. I made my escape as soon as I could, and left the room, finding an empty room nearby. Crying quietly to myself, I thought, "That was awful. I can't do this. I'll never be able to be an assistant."

A Secret Revealed
1991 (age 37)

Even though my last experience had been traumatic, I still felt drawn to the Tantra world. The freedom of sexuality enticed me, and that it was a spiritual practice. A few weeks later there was a party at the same mansion. I decided to go.

At the food table, I found myself next to a bald man with soulful brown eyes and an aura of power and masculinity.

"Hello, my name is Scott." He shook my hand while balancing a small plate of food. "My partner over there is Johanna." He pointed to a voluptuous woman with short auburn hair. "We're starting to teach Tantra too. You should come check it out."

"Maybe I will."

A week later, I made my way to their house in the suburbs. The white middle-class neighborhood seemed unlikely for Tantra. I went inside, and found a group of about twenty people sitting in a circle on the carpeted floor of a remodeled garage. Mirrors lined the walls. I found a place and settled down.

Music began, and Scott and Johanna entered, each carrying a small candle. They walked around the circle, making eye contact with each person. Once the circuit was complete, they sat in the center of the circle, facing each other. They took a few breaths together, and Johanna climbed onto Scott's lap.

A hush fell over the room as they gazed into each other's eyes. Their love for each other was palpable. I felt awe at the intensity of presence they demonstrated.

After a few moments, they moved apart and took their places in the circle. They talked about what Tantra is – the art of sacred sexuality. I had heard all that before. Then they introduced a new topic.

"Boundaries are very important when you are exploring something as intimate as Tantra," Johanna stated. "They help you feel safe enough so you can come out to play. If you don't feel safe, you'll protect yourself with a wall that keeps everyone out. You may look like you're being intimate, but you're really not even there."

I remembered leaving my body when I was assisting at the other workshop.

"There are no right answers when it comes to boundaries," Scott picked up the thread. "Whatever boundary you have is the right one for you. It's tempting to go along with what everyone else is doing so that you'll fit in, but you won't really be present if you do."

He was addressing precisely the reasons that I had done what I did – watching Hope with the ugly man and thinking that I needed to be like her.

"We're going to do an exercise now that will help you learn how to know what your boundaries are by how your body feels," Johanna continued.

I felt a growing excitement as they explained the exercise. There was something here that I really needed to learn. These people could teach me how to open to sacred sexuality in a way that didn't damage me.

I studied with Scott and Johanna for a more than two years. For most of that time, I was part of an ongoing, committed group of twenty-four people. We met once a month for a weekend each time. With that much continual exposure, we bonded deeply and built a tremendous amount of trust with each other. We shared our innermost selves as we learned how to be truly intimate.

One day the topic was seduction and how we can use it to manipulate others.

"You're really good at that, Selena," Tony said. "You do it with me all the time."

He was a muscular man with an angry edge -- a classic bad boy, just the kind of man I was most attracted to. We had flirted and enjoyed sexual energy together for the past year, when we found ourselves partnered together in the workshops. We never saw each other outside of the workshops, keeping the connection only in that sacred space.

Stricken with shame, I looked around the circle at the others. They were all smiling and nodding. I looked inward, examining my behavior. I felt a sinking feeling inside.

Summoning up courage, I spoke. "You're right. I do that. I use my sexuality to be liked, to make people feel that I'm worth something, because I'm afraid that I'm not really worth anything."

A woman across the circle spoke. "When you are honest like this, and reveal who you really are, I like you even more."

The room filled with murmurs of assent.

Tears streamed down my face as I took in what had just happened. I had revealed one of my deepest secrets to a room full of people, who loved me even more for it. Something shifted inside. If they knew this about me, and still loved me, maybe I could also love myself.

Tantra became my world, and these people my family.

5 - Building the Temple

God on his Vajra
1995 (age 41)

I bowed to Jeffrey as he entered my house. I was dressed all in white, a long dress covered by a silk robe with beads embroidered in magical symbols. He carried some blue silk boxer shorts in his hand. We walked into the healing room, and hugged each other hello.

I had been doing sexual healing work with him for about seven years. Since we lived in different states, until then we had only been able to have intermittent visits. He was here for his first weeklong intensive with me. In the past seven years we had worked extensively with building trust so that he felt safe. Both his child personality, Rusty, and the adult, Jeffrey trusted and loved me. He was ready to take a deeper step.

I lit a large white candle. "I ask for healing energies to be here with us this week. I ask that Spirit guide us, and that whatever happens here be for your highest good and light."

"We'll leave this candle burning all week," I told him. "It will keep the energy going for us."

"I've been having dreams with a goddess in them," he said as we settled down onto the sofa. "She's been telling me what to do for my healing. I'd like your help in doing the things she's told me."

"I'm happy to help," I answered. "Just tell me what you'd like."

He changed into his silk shorts, to signify that we were in ritual healing space. We sat before each other, as the goddess of his dreams had directed.

I looked into his wide innocent eyes and knew that Rusty was there. I reached out and caressed his cheek tenderly. His face crumpled and tears flowed.

"I love you, Rusty."

"Oh, I love you too," he sobbed.

Acting upon the goddess's directions, I moved my hand to his thigh. His penis stiffened instantly.

"Do you know that your vajra is erect?"

"It is?" he looked down. "No, I can't feel it."

"Feel my hand touching your vajra. I see your erection. It's good to be erect. It's a beautiful thing."

"Ohhhh . . . " He squirmed in discomfort. "My face is burning. I'm feeling shame."

"There's nothing to be ashamed of. Your vajra is beautiful. It's good to be erect. Look at my face."

He reluctantly turned back to me.

"Do I look angry?" He shook his head. "Disgusted?"

"Nooo . . . "

"It's good to be erect."

The next day, he told me of a ritual he wanted to do. He felt that there was an evil stain on his vajra. The goddess had told him to have me wash it off, and then bring God into his vajra.

He lay upon the table, naked. I brought a bowl of warm water and a washcloth and I gently washed his penis with the cloth.

"Any stain that is on your vajra is being cleansed now. This water is washing it off."

He watched me with those child-like eyes.

When I was done with the washing, I asked him to get dressed again.

"We're going to take this water and give it to the tree outside my door."

"Will it hurt the tree?" he asked in concern.

"No, trees can handle negative energy. It'll be fine."

"It was a lot of bad stuff in my vajra. Are you sure the tree will be ok?"

"Yes," I said, leading him outside. I slowly poured the bowl of water onto the roots of the big pine tree. "We give this water, and this energy taken from Jeffrey's vajra, back to this tree. We ask that it be absorbed into the earth. We ask this tree to transmute this energy into something positive, and to send it where it is needed."

The next day, he anxiously checked the pine tree.

"See, it's doing just fine," I showed him. "Let's go inside."

"Today, I want you to paint God on my vajra," he said. "I brought some body paints."

"I'd be glad to," I replied. As he undressed and got onto the table, I wondered what in the world God on a vajra would look like. I picked up a blue crayon and drew some big slanted eyes just under the head of his penis, which was erect from my touch.

"Well, that's a start," I thought to myself. "Maybe some eyebrows now." I drew a couple of black arches over the blue eyes. "It's starting to look like a face. I think its mouth should have a big smile." I traced a bright red smile under the eyes.

"God is smiling on your vajra," I told him. "See?" I held a mirror so he could look.

"God is smiling on my vajra?" he asked in disbelief.

"Yes, that's how much he likes it."

"Wow!" Rusty said.

Jeffrey was a remarkable man, and I was privileged to work with him. His guidance from the goddess in his dreams was very instrumental in his healing process. She visited him often over the next years, telling him what he needed as the next step. The rituals we did accessed a deeper part of his psyche than was possible in any other way. And it was essential that I be willing to touch his penis and to honor it, as an antidote to all the abuse he had received from his mother. In doing so, I was re-programming his sense of himself and his relationship to his penis and his sexuality.

Sensual Massage
1999 (age 45)

I. Interview

I walked into the neighborhood café, and scanned the area for the woman I was meeting. We had talked on the phone, but this was our first contact in person. I saw a woman who must have been her, sitting in a comfortable-looking armchair in a small seating area in the back of the cafe. She was about my age, mid-forties, with long red hair and pale skin, dressed casually in jeans and a sweater. As I got closer, I saw deep brown eyes that looked ancient.

"Karen?"

"Yes," she replied. "Have a seat."

I sat down a bit nervously. This was a job interview, but one that was different than any I had been to before. I was applying to work for her doing sensual massage. My income had dropped drastically recently. I needed to bring in more cash, and quickly. I had flirted with the idea of doing sensual massage for years, but always backed away. I had been scared that it would have been emotionally damaging to me, that I wouldn't be able to hold my boundaries with clients, that it would feed into my old neurosis that I was only good for one thing – sex.

Now I felt like a different person -- strong and confident, in my power. I had learned how to hold boundaries so well that I knew that I could do it in a session. And I had done enough psychological work that I knew my own worth.

Karen had been doing sensual massage herself for two years, and now she was opening her own business. She had rented a house in the neighborhood nearby, and she was ready to open it next week. She was in the process of hiring people to work there.

In our phone conversation we had talked about her other career as a psychic. As we talked about the job, I was aware that we were both studying each other closely. I liked what I saw. She had a direct gaze, with no nervous shifting of eyes. She spoke honestly of the range of experience that sensual massage could bring.

"Most of the clients are really sweet," she said. "I like them a lot. Then there are some who are challenging. Some will push your boundaries, and try to sneak a hand where you don't want it. Some have smelly butt cracks. But all in all, I like it a lot."

"How does a session go?"

"Well, I usually start off with offering them a shower and taking their money, then I leave the room. When I come back they are lying face down on the table. As soon as I've closed the door, I take my dress off. They think it's seductive, but it's really to keep the oil stains off my dress. Then I give them about a half-hour massage on their backs and legs. I end it with tickling their balls and getting them a little worked up. Then I ask them to turn over, and I take off my lingerie."

"Is there anything special I should wear?"

"Whatever makes you look good."

"So then what?"

"Different people do it different ways. Some people stand beside the table and give them a hand job. I like to climb up on the table with them, and rub my body against theirs. Whatever you do is fine. Most people let the clients fondle their breasts and suck on them."

I digested this information. How would it feel to do this with a perfect stranger? I didn't know. I felt excited and nervous all at the same time.

"OK, I think I'd like to try it," I said.

"Great! I'd love to have you there. Can you start next week?"

We worked out the details, and parted with a hug. I trusted this woman.

II. The First Days
I spent the weekend shopping for dresses and lingerie. I didn't have anything that seemed suitable, and I wanted to have clothing that was only for work, so it would be like putting on a different persona. I wanted a different name as well. I pondered this for days. One day in yoga class, I was doing a posture called *ardachandrasana* – half moon pose. I had it! I would call myself Chandra, which means moon. It was perfect. I was so connected with the moon, and I liked having a Sanskrit name since I was promoting myself as a Tantrika.

My first day at work was the first day Karen opened her business. No one knew we were there yet, so business was very slow. I spent the day sitting around the table with the other women, getting to know them and the space. I was content to just be there, and ease slowly into the environment. After a while, I grew restless, and asked Karen if she needed any help, as she was still settling into the house. She asked me to clean the moldings around the walls. As I worked, we talked and laughed.

"Hey! I'm doing the *other* traditional women's work now – cleaning the house," I joked.

The next day that I worked, I heard Karen making an appointment for me. I felt a rush of excitement and nervousness in my chest.

"He's coming in half an hour. Don't let him know that you're new. Some men will try to take advantage of the new ones."

"OK," I said, wide-eyed. How would someone take advantage of me? Run all over me? Inwardly, I gulped.

I prepared for my client, dressing in my new pink dress with the hearts on it. I brushed my hair, and put lipstick on. I had to wipe it off and try again because I was so inexperienced with makeup. Even so, I was ready soon, and waiting for him to show up.

I heard a knock on the door, and opened it to find a short, chubby man with curly brown hair. He was not much taller than me. He didn't look so threatening. I welcomed him inside, and led him back to the room, where soft music was playing. I took his money, and invited him to lie upon the table while I left the room.

When I walked back into the room, I felt uncomfortable, knowing that Karen had said that she took her dress off as soon as she got into the room. I didn't feel ready to do that, so I decided to wait. After all, he was face down. He couldn't see me anyway. I gave myself the time.

I was used to giving a massage that lasted at least an hour, and usually an hour and a half, so I was not quite sure of my timing yet. When I asked him to turn over, he looked up and said "So soon?"

I looked at the clock and saw that it had only been twenty minutes. Ooops! I gave him a little more back massage, then again asked him to turn over. He looked at me, and I slowly pulled my dress over my head, still leaving my white lace teddy on. "OK, I did it." I thought. "I undressed in front of him. That wasn't so bad."

I began to feel more relaxed and comfortable. I lightly stroked his body, playing with the hair on his chest and legs. I slipped the straps off my shoulders so that one breast was exposed, then the other. He reached up and cupped my breast in his hand. I leaned down so that he could suckle the nipple, while my hand reached out to fondle his cock. After a few moments, he tensed and ejaculated.

"Wow! That was fast." I thought to myself. "No wonder he was concerned about it being so soon when I asked him to turn over."

I went and got a warm wet washcloth and gently cleaned him up. I offered him more massage, but he declined. We both got dressed and I saw him out.

"My first session! I did it!" I crowed to the others. "It was fine!"

"Yes, and you made $100 in less than an hour," Karen reminded me. "I booked another one for you while you were in there. He's coming in fifteen minutes."

"Yikes! Let me get ready," I exclaimed. I ran to change the sheets on the table, and then came back to brush my hair and straighten my dress. I had a couple of minutes to spare, and the next client arrived.

The next session proceeded much like the first, although I was much more comfortable this time. Again, I allowed him to kiss my breasts and suck on my nipples. He was good at it. As I stood there beside him, pleasuring his penis as he pleasured my breasts, I felt myself getting aroused. It dawned on me – this was allowed! For so long I had been doing sexual healing work. It was serious, often working with deep trauma, and I had the responsibility of holding the container for the client. It was about her or him, not about me and my pleasure. Now I was in a totally different situation. These clients didn't need me to hold back my own feelings. They probably would like it better if I didn't.

Leaning over his face, rubbing my breasts all over him, being caressed skillfully, I felt my excitement building until an orgasm overtook me. Still we continued touching each other, and soon I had another orgasm. This time he came with me.

After he left, I walked back into the break room where the other women waited. My face was glowing.

"Looks like you had a good time," Karen commented.

"I had two orgasms," I said, still slightly amazed that this was my new job. "I was made to do this work!"

Soon the house became known. Clients flocked to our doors, and I was seeing four, five, and even six people per day. I flowed from one session to another, often in a constant state of arousal. Some days I felt like I was in a day-long orgasm. I loved each day.

Even while enjoying the work so much, I had to readjust my attitudes about myself in relationship to society. I would look at the people in the grocery store and wonder what they would think of me if they knew what I was doing. I felt at odds with the mainstream, vulnerable to censure for something that I valued so highly. Luckily, I had the other women with whom I worked, as well as friends who accepted and approved of what I was doing.

I walked into work one morning to find Alexandria already there. She was a petite woman with wild brown curls and large round blue eyes.

"Hi, ho!" she greeted me. Then she whispered, "Say it back."

Somewhat bewildered, I replied, "Hi, ho."

"It's off to work we go!" She sang. We both laughed.

One Saturday morning, a day that we were closed for clients, we all had a meeting. I met some of the women who worked on different days for the first time. Karen brought bagels and other food, and spread out a simple feast. The talk was lively, and I was impressed with the vivaciousness of these beautiful women. There were no victims here. Each woman was there by choice, and feeling positive about what she was doing.

Lilah, a beautiful Latina woman with sparkling eyes and a curvy figure, spoke to Karen. "You've created a wonderful place here. It's different than any other place that I've worked. I feel relaxed and at home here. You take such good care of us, and you've attracted amazing people to work here."

A round of assents supported her statement. Karen turned away for a moment, then faced us again, tears in her eyes. "It's why I did this. I want this to be a place that will support you, help you make good money, and help you realize whatever your dreams are."

We all came together in a hug.

Addiction
1999 (age 45)

I opened the door to admit my last client of the day. A very short man with metal crutches stood on the porch. His large upper body was incongruous with his small legs. He was impeccably dressed in a beige linen jacket and a silk shirt, and he looked ill at ease. I hid my surprise and invited him in. He followed me into the candle-lit room, and dropped down on the sofa with relief.

"Can we take care of the financial part first?" I asked him.

"I'd like a sample of your touch," Joseph countered.

Taken aback, I thought rapidly. It was my first week of sensual massage work and I was still unsure of myself. "What should I do here? How should I handle this?" I took a breath to center myself and sat beside him. I put my hand on his knee. His leg was atrophied. "Oh, no, maybe I shouldn't have done that. Maybe he's self-conscious about his leg," I second-guessed myself. Nevertheless, I left my hand there, stayed calm, and sent caring energy through my hand. We sat in silence.

"All right," he said. "I'll give you the money."

When I returned from taking care of the money, he was still sitting there.

"Would you like to get undressed and on the table?" I invited.

He glanced at the height of the table. "No, I'll just sit here."

I knelt on the floor in front of him and placed my hands on his legs, sliding them up his thighs to his hips. I looked into his beautiful brown eyes with kindness. "What would you like?"

"Stroke me in a way that will arouse me."

This session was different than the few I had experienced so far, in which I would give the client a back massage while he was face down for the first thirty minutes. I could use that time to get comfortable before the session moved into more erotic touch. But in this session that time was not available. I took another deep breath, and caressed his legs through his pants.

After a few moments, he was ready to take them off. I assisted him, finding leather braces around both his legs. Removing them was a lengthy process. He was very precise in his movements, putting his braces aside with the fasteners lined up beside each other. After the braces were placed, he took off his jacket and shirt, folding them neatly, and sat there again wearing just his white tank-top undershirt. His chest was broad and tanned, with white hair peeking above the undershirt. His pale legs were small and weak.

As I knelt in front of him again, I felt myself become a channel for the goddess. I could see how much he needed love, and how scared, insecure, and vulnerable he was. Words started pouring out of my mouth. "You deserve to be pleasured. You deserve lots of love. I want you to feel as much pleasure as you possibly can."

"Oh, Chandra!" he sighed. I smiled to myself, still not used to the name. "Chandra, I want you to make me addicted to you."

A tiny flag raised, but I brushed it aside. I caressed him gently. "Breathe in this love that is flowing through me. Bring it into your heart. It is from the goddess."

He sighed and moaned in pleasure, and soon orgasmed.

"Oh, Chandra," he marveled. "I never expected anything like this. Thank you."

The next week he came back. Again the genuine words of love poured through me. It was as if I were a fountain of goddess energy. "Here is love, drink from it. Drink from it."

He asked me to put a finger in his anus. Slowly and gently I obliged. His pleasure was even deeper this time than before.

A month went by before he returned.

"I felt really guilty after the last session."

"What for?" I asked.

"The anal stuff. It's not natural."

"Not natural?"

"Yes, it's not the natural order of things. Sex is supposed to be about a penis being in a vagina. It's deviant – perverted – to enjoy anal sex like I do."

"You do enjoy it?" I asked. He nodded. "Then it's a wonderful thing. Bodies are to be enjoyed. The way I see it, God wouldn't have made our bodies capable of having pleasure if we weren't supposed to have it."

"My father told me long ago that I shouldn't get into doing anything with my ass. He said it would be opening Pandora's box."

"Would you like some help with changing this attitude?" I asked him.

"It's not an attitude, Chandra, it's just the truth."

"Look, there's something that you like a lot, that you feel terribly guilty about when you do it. I think I can help you accept it more easily. Would you like my help?"

He hesitated. "Yes," he said.

Our sessions fell into a pattern. We spent the first half hour with my pleasuring him, mostly anally, and then we would talk together. He told me that I was more effective than any psychologist he had engaged. He often visited me weekly. Occasionally a month would go by, because he felt so guilty and ashamed of himself. I tried to get him to come regularly so that we could address those feelings, but he was resistant.

He often expressed fear that he was a sex addict. He told me of ruining a relationship because he couldn't stop going to prostitutes. He felt out of control, and at the mercy of his addiction.

"I'm addicted to you, Chandra," he said.

"I only want to see you if it is in your best interest. If it's causing you conflict in your life, then don't come and see me."

He took a deep breath. "I'm not going to see you anymore."

It was a fine line I was walking. I was trying to help him reframe his attitudes about his sexuality, but I was growing discouraged with his lack of change. I was becoming more and more concerned about his addictive behavior.

The next week he was back.

"Chandra, will you marry me? You could keep working, and I'd give you a great place to live."

"No, Joseph, I won't marry you. These sessions are all we'll ever have."

Disappointed, he asked, "Please pleasure me."

A few months later, he said for the umpteenth time, "This is going to be the last time."

Silently, I said, "Yeah, right, sure. You've said that before."

"But I don't want to talk about it," he continued.

"All right," I agreed, and began pleasuring him.

The next week, he didn't call. Weeks went by, and finally the phone rang. It was Joseph.

"I've been abstinent for two months now. I'm feeling really good about myself. It was really hard. Sometimes I felt like crawling the walls. It would have been so easy to call you but I really wanted to break the addiction."

"Good for you!" I said. "I'm so happy for you. It's a great thing that you are doing, and it took a lot of discipline. I'm proud of you."

"Will you call me some time?"

"No, I won't. I want to support you in keeping with this. You're doing a good thing."

He never called back.

I thought I could help this man embrace his sexual preferences and let go of his self-judgments, but I was never able to. His mind was so firmly set that it refused to change. Eventually, I realized that it would serve him more to just let him go. He was not really open for deeper healing.

Therapeutic Meets Sensual
2000 (age 46)

"I have an enlarged prostate, and my doctor told me to get prostate massage," he said on the phone. "Can you help me? I don't know where else to go to get it."

"I certainly can," I assured him. "I've done lots of prostate massages. You've chosen a good person to do it."

"Do you use gloves?" he asked nervously.

I smiled to myself. He was not sure what to expect. Perhaps he was wondering if the experience would be dirty or unsafe. He probably had the typical cultural stereotypes of what prostitution is about.

"I use the same kind of gloves that doctors do."

"Ok, let's book a session."

When he arrived, he was a little edgy. A tall man with dark hair, he was middle-aged and looked middle class, like most of my clients, if he had only known.

"I'm really not looking for a sexual experience. I really do want a therapeutic prostate massage," he asserted.

"That's fine with me," I told him. "Whatever you want."

I invited him to lie face down on the table, and proceeded to give him a deep therapeutic massage on his back, legs, and buttocks. I knew that if he was relaxed that the prostate massage would go much more easily. His body softened under my touch.

When I invited him to turn over, he stirred slowly. "Wow, I know that I'm in good hands!"

I smiled at him, and pulled on a glove. "I'm going to start by massaging your perineum before I go inside to get to your prostate. It will help you to open up more. Please let me know if anything doesn't feel comfortable. We'll go slowly so you have time to open."

I coated my finger with lubricant, and began to massage firmly on his perineum. He let go even more deeply.

"Now let me begin to touch your anus to help it open. I won't go inside unless I get your permission. Is that ok?"

"Yes, that's fine. This is really different than how the doctor does it."

"I have a friend who is a medical doctor. He told me that they teach them in medical school to be rough while doing prostate exams, so that people don't confuse it with sexuality. Isn't that barbaric?"

He nodded and agreed.

I began to stroke around his anus, using firm pressure to stretch the muscles open. I let the tip of my finger go inside his anus just a little.

"I call this knocking at the door," I told him. "I'm just letting your body know that I'm there, and when you are ready, you can invite me inside."

"I think I'm ready," he said.

I applied more lubricant to my finger, and pressed it up against his anus.

"Take a deep breath in," I directed him. As he did, the natural relaxation of the pelvic muscles allowed my finger to sink inside a little more. "Do that again."

Working with his breath, I slowly penetrated him until my finger was all the way inside. I reached upwards toward his belly and felt the hard smoothness of his prostate.

"I feel it now. Yes, it is enlarged. Can you feel me touching it?"

"Yes, it feels a little strange, but it's ok," he replied.

I began moving my finger in long slow strokes across the length of his prostate. Suddenly he got an erection.

"Wow! This has never happened before," he said with some embarrassment.

"It's perfectly natural," I reassured him. "It's an area that is very pleasurable if it's touched right. Would you like me to pleasure your cock too while I do this? It will help you release even more deeply."

"Yes, that would be really good." His pelvis began to move in pleasure.

I continued the prostate massage while I began caressing his penis with my other hand. He was oozing lots of prostatic fluid as he thrashed around the table. I followed his movements. Soon his excitement built up and he ejaculated.

"That was really wonderful," he thanked me. "I never expected that it would be so pleasurable."

"I'm glad you came to me for this," I told him. "I'm comfortable with sexual energy, and I believe that it benefits your prostate more when you let it flow. If you had done this in a clinical setting, your therapist would have been really uncomfortable with your erection and it would have been a very awkward situation for both of you. This is much healthier for you."

Heart Energy
2002 (age 48)

I lay on the table with Dan, snuggled into his arm with my head on his shoulder. We were at the end of a sensual massage session, and both of us were relaxed with a post-orgasmic glow. He was someone I had seen many times over the course of the past three years. He was a middle-aged man, average in every way, but he was easy to be with and we had a mutual respect for each other.

As I rested there, I began to notice that my heart felt lonely. It didn't fit the situation. I was very connected to him. We had just experienced a great deal of passion with each other. Naked on the table together, he had climbed on top of me at my invitation. Always conscious of safer sex practices, I had kept a firm hold on his penis so that it would not enter me or touch my mucus membranes, but we had writhed together sensually as if we were making love, and we both had exploded in orgasm just a few minutes before.

I remembered his words just before he came. "Oh, Chandra . . . I give myself to you. I give you my energy, I give you my sperm, I give you my money. You receive it all."

"Yes, Dan, I receive *you.*" With these words, he had slid into orgasm.

Now, I realized that it wasn't my heart that was lonely, it was his. I remembered his wedding ring, and the wife that we never mentioned.

"Is your heart lonely, Dan?" I dared to ask.

He looked away, and I saw a tear in the corner of his eye. I stroked his hair, his cheek.

"It's ok, you can tell me about it if you want," I soothed him.

The story that I had already guessed came pouring out. The cold marriage, the wife not interested in sex. Living a life without affection. Staying together because of the kids. The house in the suburbs. The dreary responsibility.

"I'm basically a monogamous man," he said. "These days, I'm monogamous with you."

"I'm glad that I can be here for you," I said. Inwardly I was gulping in dismay. I saw him only about every six weeks. What a long time to go between moments of affection! I cuddled in closer. "You deserve a lot of love. You're such a good man."

"I remember the first session we had," he said to me. "You won my heart that day."

"How did I do that?"

"I was lying on the table, on my back. You took your clothes off and climbed up on the table and kneeled above me. When I came, you were rubbing my cock all over your breasts. The semen covered you. Instead of wiping it off, you just rubbed it into your skin, and you said, 'I'm rubbing this into my heart'. I just melted then."

I smiled, remembering the moment. "That was great. I loved doing that."

"Then you thanked me for the gift of my semen. I couldn't believe it."

"It *is* a gift. It's your life force essence. It's full of energy and light."

Many of the sensual massage clients were married men, trying to stay faithful in marriages that didn't include sex or intimacy. Often they valued their wives as friends, partners and co-parents, but the lack of sexuality left a dilemma. What were they supposed to do with their sexual energy? There were no good choices. They could shut it down and loose their vitality. They could have an affair and risk the emotional entanglements that could mean the end of their marriage. Many chose another option – to receive sensual massage. By the nature of its business arrangement, neither party was interested in further emotional involvement. Perhaps they rationalized that since our sessions didn't include intercourse that they weren't really breaking any agreements. This was a way to find an outlet for their sexual energy. I imagined that they would go home to their wives with a little less tension, and perhaps be nicer to them without all that need behind their actions.

Making Love to Yourself
2001 (age 47)

He was a tow truck driver, sloppy fat with greasy hair and black under his fingernails. His shirttail hung out on one side, and his khaki pants were baggy.

Inwardly revolted, I welcomed him in. Remembering my ethic of finding something loveable about each person, I softened as I gazed at him.

"How may I serve you?"

"I've heard that Tantra will help me slow down. I could use that."

"Yes, I can teach you a way to breathe that will help you with that."

At my direction, he started face down on the table. I massaged his back and legs, using deep firm strokes. His body gradually loosened up, and he sank into a profound state of relaxation.

After about half an hour, I asked him to turn over. Slowly, he complied, murmuring, "That was great."

"I'm so glad. Let me tell you now about how to delay ejaculation."

His eyes focused more clearly on me, and I began to explain the mechanics of drawing energy up the spine away from the pelvis. I asked him to tell me when he needed to slow down, so I could help him redistribute the energy.

Once he was familiar with the process of delay, I encouraged him to just lie back and enjoy the touch. Caressing him lightly on his legs and thighs stimulated an erection almost immediately. I stroked around his lingam, not touching it, and moved up his belly and chest with my hands. After a few minutes of teasing him, I took his penis in my hands and held it gently.

"Remember, tell me when you want to slow down."

"All right. It feels really good."

I poured some lubricant into my hands and enjoyed the slippery feel as my hands slid all over his lingam. Suddenly his body tensed and his eyes grew wide.

"Whoa! Slow down!" Instantly I stopped, but it was too late. His cock twitched and semen began to flow.

"Just let go and enjoy," I encouraged. "Don't try to stop it now." I knew that if he did, he would still have the ejaculation, but no orgasm or pleasure.

As his orgasm subsided, I glanced at the clock. It had been five minutes since I had begun touching him. "Wow, he really does need some help," I thought to myself. "I had no idea how trigger-happy he was."

"This is just part of the learning process," I told him once he was able to hear me again. "You have to learn your body to be able to do this technique. That's the tricky part. It takes practice. The more you practice, the more you will begin to know when you are getting close, and you can slow down sooner. Practice makes perfect!"

"Should I come to see you again?" he asked.

"Yes, I'd be happy to help you practice," I answered. "And you can also practice with yourself. Make love to yourself, and practice delaying. You'll learn a lot."

"Make love to myself? You mean masturbate?"

"Yes, I like to call it making love to myself. It has a whole different feel than the word masturbation. Masturbation sounds like something dirty, something you do as quickly as possible so you won't get caught. That's why a lot of men have trouble with premature ejaculation. As teenagers they trained themselves to come as fast as they could, hiding in the bathroom."

"Yes, I did that."

"So now you can train yourself differently. Set it up as a ritual. Light candles, be in front of a mirror. Pleasure yourself while looking into your own eyes. Tell yourself 'I love you.' Celebrate yourself."

"That's really different than anything I've ever done."

"Yes, I'm sure it is. Does it sound like fun?"

"Yes, it does," he said, his eyes wandering off in contemplation.

"The Buddha said that you can travel the world over and never find another person more deserving of love than you. This is a way to express that."

One of the pleasures of doing sensual massage was that I reached people who would never have come to see me if I had called my work "spiritual" or "healing". Yet often they were the ones most in need of healing. The promise of an exotic sexual experience lured them in, and once they were there, they often received much more than just a hand job. Like with this man, I used the opening that happened with orgasm as a way in, to plant seeds of self-loving, heart-healing, and a glimpse of a broader reality.

Just Having Fun
2000 (age 46)

"Can Tantra help me with erectile dysfunction?" Robert asked, as he clasped his hands and leaned forward.

This was our first session. He was an older man, with white hair and saggy muscles. His blue eyes looked at me hopefully.

"Well, there are a lot of reasons for that, so it can be complicated. Let's start with the easiest ones first – the physical causes. Have you seen a doctor about this?"

"Yes, he didn't find anything wrong."

"Do you smoke?"

"No," he answered.

"Good. Smoking will constrict the blood flow to the penis and make it harder to have an erection. How much exercise do you get?"

"Well, I don't do very much."

"You might try adding some aerobic exercise to your daily routine. If you have good circulation, then you're more likely to get good blow flow."

I continued to ask him questions about his physical health – diabetes, antidepressants, and his general health condition.

Nothing seemed to be out of the ordinary, so I moved into another area.

"Sometimes when you focus upon trying to get an erection too much, it actually gets in the way. You give yourself performance pressure. When you think to yourself, 'I wonder if I'll stay soft this time,' your brain hears 'stay soft' and it cooperates."

He chuckled a little. "Yes, I can see that."

"One thing that Tantra teaches is to just stay in the moment, without an agenda of what *should* happen. You can enjoy the sensations of sexual touch whether you have an erection or not. If you're working hard to have an erection, then sex becomes work, not fun. And isn't it supposed to be fun?"

"Yes, I guess it is."

"So let's try a little experiment. Let me pleasure you, and instead of trying to make something happen, let yourself just have fun."

"Ok," he agreed. "Sounds good to me."

As I touched him, I made sure to include his whole body, with only incidental touches to his lingam. I made my pace leisurely, reminding him from time to time to focus just upon the touch in the moment without needing it to go anywhere next. His body responded to my touch with relaxation, and he began to drift.

Soon, his penis began to enlarge. I began to focus more upon it, adding lubricant to make a sensuous slippery feel. His mouth opened in arousal and his lingam got harder.

"Oh, that feels good," he breathed.

"Good, I'm glad you're enjoying it. Just continue to pay attention to each touch, as if you have never been touched before. Notice how it is different one moment to the next."

I encircled the base of his penis with my thumb and fingers, trapping the blood and creating a full erection. My other hand continued to glide over his lingam.

"Oh! I'm going to come!" he exclaimed.

"Good, let yourself do that," I purred.

His body stiffened and his face reddened as he ejaculated. Soon, he collapsed into a complete relaxation. Moments passed in silence as I continued to cup his genitals in my hands.

"Thank you so much." He slowly opened his eyes and looked at me. "It's been a really long time since that happened."

"See what happens when you drop the goal and stay in the moment?" I smiled at him. "Did you have fun?"

"Yes, it was great fun! Much better than working at it," he laughed.

"Now you know what is possible. You can do this again."

Priestess Reborn
1999 (age 45)

"Can you find me a sex surrogate to work with?" Jeffrey asked in a phone call. "The goddess in my dreams is telling me I need to do that. I tried one, but she was awful. She got on top of me and kept telling me I should thrust; that women like that. I was really scared. I got frozen."

I paused for a moment, trying to think if there was anyone I knew who would be able to approach him with the gentleness that he needed. I drew a blank. There was no one who had the kind of sensitivity that I had used with him over the years. No one but me.

"No one comes to mind right away, but I'll think about it," I promised him, and hung up.

Could I do it? I had never done anything remotely like that before. I had always kept myself strictly separate from my healing clients, even while giving them sexual touch as part of their healing process. I could see the value in it for him. I knew that he trusted me, and that I would be more successful in his healing process than most anyone I could imagine.

But what if I said I would and then I wasn't turned on? What if my own issues of performance pressure got activated? If I were not able to follow through, it would be devastating for him. He would assume that it was because there was something wrong with him, no matter how much I tried to reassure him differently.

I prayed and meditated, asking Spirit for guidance. The answer I got was to do it.

"Can you go really slow?" he asked me. "The energy gets so big that it's overwhelming to me. I need to do it a little at a time."

"Yes, I'd be happy to go slow. That works for me too."

He was lying on the massage table, naked with a sheet over him. I stood beside him, with my arms around him. I was still clothed. He was somewhat agitated, nervous about what we were going to do. I focused upon soothing him, stroking him slowly and lovingly, and speaking softly to him.

"Whatever happens is fine. We can stop at any time." I was saying this as much to myself as to him. I was afraid that I would freeze, that I wouldn't be able to be there for him because I was too wrapped up in having to perform. It was a delicate situation. I had such a strong habit of not reacting sexually to him, and now I needed to undo it. Not only that, but I knew that at any moment he could have some kind of emotional reaction and I would need to be completely present. There would be no abandonment into my feelings for me that day.

"Would you like me to take my clothes off now?" I asked. He nodded, and I pulled my dress over my head. I had chosen a turquoise silk camisole and boy shorts, wanting to be dressed sensually but not too blatantly erotic. I removed the underwear, and stood there beside him again.

"Can I get on the table with you?" I asked. When he agreed, I climbed up and snuggled in beside him. I caressed his chest and belly with my free hand, and he began to be aroused.

"Is this ok?" I asked.

"Yes, it feels good."

"Let me know anytime you feel scared or ashamed. We can stop anytime and work with what you're feeling." I continued to stroke him, my hand moving lower towards his groin.

"Ohhhh . . ." he moaned. "There's a lot of energy." His brow furrowed.

"It's ok to have the energy. You're safe. Remember that it's me."

"Ok."

I touched him some more, and his penis grew even harder. "Can I put the condom on you now?"

"Yes."

I slowly unrolled the condom over his lingam. "Can I get on top of you?"

"Yes, I'd like that."

I reached one leg over him and moved up so that his penis was just at the opening of my vagina. "I'm going to wait here. Just feel the energy of my yoni. How does it feel?"

"It feels good."

"Good." I moved a little so that the tip of his penis touched the most sensitive places of my yoni. I could feel myself moistening. A kind of a calm descended over me. I felt myself alight with the ancient lineage of sexual healers, and my ego became insignificant. It didn't matter whether I was attracted to him or not. My body was in service to the goddess, and the goddess was serving him. My yoni opened and softened.

"Are you ready to enter me?" I asked.

"Yes, please go slow," he implored me. "It's really intense."

"I'll go as slow as you like." I slid down over his erect penis a millimeter at a time, watching his face carefully for reactions. An expression of bliss crossed over him, and I relaxed slightly. He was doing well, and so was I.

"Oh! It's so good! I can't believe how good it is!" he exclaimed.

"Yes, it is. Can you take it if I let a little more energy out?"

"Yes! Oh, yes, I'd like that."

I gradually modulated my arousal higher, paying close attention to his reactions. He was doing fine, enjoying himself. I let myself get more passionate. He put his arms around me, with his eyes closed and a heavenly smile on his face.

My excitement grew until my body rippled in an orgasm. I cried out, and his pelvis thrust upward to reach deeper inside me.

I slowed my movements, and quickly asked, "How are you?"

"I'm ok," he replied. "I don't think I can come inside you though."

"Why not?"

"It would slime you."

"Oh, honey, you won't slime me. But if you'd like me to get off you now and pleasure you with my hand, I'd be glad to do that. Maybe you've had enough for today."

"Yes, I think so."

I slid off him and removed the condom. Filling my hand with lubricant, I gently stroked him until he ejaculated.

"You did so well today, Jeffrey! That was a lot. You did great!"

My fears of not being aroused were coming from my personal self, my ego. Before the session, I had thought that *I* would be doing the session. During the session it became clear that all I needed to do was to get out of the way and let the goddess work through me. Once I connected with my self as priestess, it was effortless to be sexual with him. I was in service to him, and through him to all the people wounded in the area of sexuality. It was bigger than Selena and Jeffrey. Our interaction was timeless, one in a string of holy connections throughout the ages. The sacred prostitute was reborn in me that day.

Darkness
2002 (age 48)

It was a hard day for me. I had not slept much for several days. My mother had just told me that morning that she might have congestive heart failure. I had clients scheduled back to back. Phil was the third.

As the day went on, I realized that I was in no shape to see him. He was a small, groveling man, with brown eyes magnified by his glasses. I had seen him once before. In our previous session, he had wanted me to inflict pain upon him. He took my hands and pushed my fingernails into his nipples with all his strength. Since then, he had left a couple of phone messages, with an underlying tone of obsession. I had no patience for his fantasies, his desire to be dominated and humiliated. There was no part of me that could relate to that, nor did I want to.

I left a message for him to call me before he came. When he called, he was almost to my place, with only about a half-hour before our appointment time. I could hear that he was in his car as we talked. I knew that he had come from a distance, and that he had been looking forward to our appointment since we had made it a couple of weeks before. I told him that I was not interested in role-play or fantasy, and he agreed. He asked if he could still come to see me and even though my instincts said not to see him, I agreed out of a sense of obligation.

He arrived shortly thereafter. We talked for a while. He explained that pain takes him to a higher place. As he talked,

113

I could relate to what he was saying. I asked him to focus not on surrender to me, but to surrender to the energy, and I agreed to do the session.

I began the session with soft touch, first on his back, then on the front of his body. I began to linger on his nipples. Knowing how much pain would send him into an altered state, I began to squeeze his nipples harder. I had experienced for myself the ecstasy that pain brings, and I understood the surrender involved.

He reached for my hands, and positioned my fingernails over his nipples. He pushed them into his nipples, and I saw him arch his back and sharply inhale. He continued to push my fingernails into his nipples, going deeper and deeper into the pain.

Then he took my left hand and moved it to his penis. He placed my hand so that my fingernail was at the tip of his urethra, then pushed it in as hard as he could. He again arched and moaned.

I felt myself begin to dissociate. I felt disoriented, dizzy, and slightly nauseous. We continued for a while, and then I finally said, "I can't do this anymore. I can't inflict pain upon you. I'm too much of an empath."

Again he talked about how pain takes him to a place of surrender, to a higher place. He spoke about how much power is in my fingertips.

I said to him, "Let me use my power more subtly. Let me use light touch with you."

He agreed. Then he reached up to my third eye with two fingers, quickly touched me there, and moved his fingers.

The rest of the session is somewhat hazy for me. I became more and more spacey, and not really in my body. I know that I touched his root chakra with my right fingertips and his lingam with my left, running energy between them.

At one point, as I stood beside him on the table, he reached behind me and touched my low back, just to the side of my spine. Another time he touched my sacrum. As he touched me, my energy began spinning upward, and I let it run. I felt confused. I knew that he was powerful energetically. I could feel how he was affecting me as he touched me, and I didn't know whether to trust him.

As the session went on, he put nipple clamps on himself, very strong ones. He knelt on the table as I stood beside it, masturbating himself as I touched his root chakra. I became more and more dissociated, until I was just enduring the session. He finally orgasmed that way, and the session was over.

I was very quiet as he got dressed and told me what a wonderful session it was.

After he left, I cried and cried, with all the stresses of the day converging.

The next day, I went out to the mountains with a friend. Again I cried, sobbing with all my being for at least an hour straight. Toward the end, I felt him again. I realized how he had hooked me energetically. I started getting him out, yelling with all my might, "No! No! No!" I used my hand to pull him out of me, out of my third eye, out of my yoni, out of my belly. I shook him out of my hands. I expelled him with righteous anger.

As I thought more about what had happened, it became clear to me. The dark forces were using him. I was under attack. I saw the remnants of light in him, and I was attracted to offering healing to him. But was too late for him. He had been taken by the dark for his whole lifetime. My guess is that he had an abusive childhood, and that had broken him. That had left the opening for the dark to come in and use him. At the same time he was powerful and adept at energy. He saw the power that I held and he wanted to use it. He corded me first at my third eye, which was my strongest point. I lost my ability to see what was happening. He then used my power to add to his.

I resolved to never see him again.

One of the challenges with sensual massage work was that I never knew who would walk through my door. Perhaps it would be someone like Phil, although he was an extreme example. It could be a man who would challenge my boundaries and make me assert myself. It could be someone lonely who would cord me unconsciously out of living an isolated life. It could be an undercover policeman, hoping to arrest me. Most often it was a sweetheart, someone who was balanced and joyful in his sexuality and who energized me as much as I energized them.

Since our culture is so sex-negative, the sexual nature of the sessions could bring out anything – guilt, shame, desire, obsession, pain. Usually the client would not even be aware of all this, and sometimes it could be projected upon me instead.

It was a delicate balance with a new client. I had to be able to rapidly assess who he was and decide how much I could open and be vulnerable, and how much I should protect myself. The fact that what I was doing was illegal meant that I couldn't talk openly about what the session would be like, in case the client was an undercover policeman with a tape recorder. This meant that I started the session without the benefit of talking frankly with the client about what he needed – unlike

116

any other therapeutic situation. I sometimes felt that I was shooting in the dark.

I developed a very fine attunement with my intuition. I could usually tell within the first few seconds of a phone call how the session would be, and I was usually right.

Occasionally I was wrong. If I was, I usually erred on the side of being too open. There was a price for that. I found that I needed to clear my energy often, and even so, it was challenging to keep it clear. Sometimes I would be weighed down with pain not my own, and I would need to cry it out or scream it out. I felt as if that was part of my service to the world, to transmute The Pain – pain that is universal.

Baptism
2003 (age 49)

The sun-warmed white granite boulders rose in sensual rounded shapes on both sides of the large green pool in the river. The water beckoned after a long hot walk. Jeffrey and I stripped our clothes off and plunged into the silky cool water.

He was visiting me for a weeklong private intensive. As we walked I had reflected upon the change in him since the last intensive several years before when I painted "God" on his vajra. He was mostly integrated now, the two personalities blended to produce a man who had a sense of humor and showed much more expression on his face. The wounding in his sexuality was still there, but not as severe. Today we wanted to address shame.

We swam and played in the river for a while, enjoying the moment. The rocks were warm, and we went in and out of the water, alternately getting cold and hot. But there were others here at this popular nude beach, so I suggested that we move upstream.

As we slowly made our way, I thought to myself how much this river was like the emotions that we experience in our lives. In places the water was shallow and we waded easily. Other times, we had to fight our way through rapids, moving against the strong current with the single-pointed goal of reaching the next rock. There were calm pools through which we gracefully swam, and small rapids where we stopped to play like children on a merry-go-round.

At last we reached a quiet pool. No one else would disturb us there, because it was so difficult to reach. Large boulders protected us, standing in the middle of the river on the upstream end of the pool. The canyon walls were steep and narrow, giving the space definition. Smaller boulders screened the downstream end of the pool. It felt safe.

"This is it," I announced to Jeffrey. "Where would you like to be?"

"How about over there?" he pointed to a flat rock about the size of a bed nestled between a couple of boulders that towered over it.

"Great choice!" I agreed. We swam across the deep still pool and climbed up onto the warm surface of the rock.

"This is what I want to do," I said to him. "I want to pleasure you here, and when you start feeling the shame come up, jump into the river and let it be washed away."

"Ok," he said a little hesitantly.

He stretched out on the rock and I sat at his side. I began to stroke his large pale body, still covered with droplets of water that glistened in the sun. He responded quickly, and began to quiver.

"Are you feeling shame?" I asked.

"Yes," he whispered.

"Let it build more before you jump," I instructed him.

I began to get more erotic in my touch, moving closer to his groin in my pathway up and down his body. His lingam stiffened and twitched.

"Oh!" he drew out the word anxiously. His face furrowed in concern.

"It's ok, let the shame come up even more," I encouraged. I held his lingam. "Do you see me holding your vajra?"

"Yes," he whimpered. "Oh . . . " He was in distress.

"Do you feel shame?"

"Yes." His head turned from side to side, as if he wanted to avoid being seen.

"Then jump into the water now," I urged. "Wash all this shame away. It doesn't belong to you."

He stood up at the edge of the rock, penis erect, and plunged into the pool. I followed, and joined him as he surfaced.

"How do you feel?" I asked him.

"Great!" he said excitedly.

"Then let's go over to that rock," I said. "I want to pleasure you with no shame."

We swam to a rock in the middle of the pool. It was the most exposed place in our whole little area, a site that shame would not have chosen. We clambered up and he reclined on his back. Again, I sat beside him. I slowly and gently caressed him with my hand, smiling at him in celebration. He gave himself over to the sensations, surrendering into the experience. His body shuddered with kundalini as the intensity grew until finally he ejaculated onto his belly.

"Does it smell bad?" he asked me with concern.

"No, it smells normal," I assured him.

"My semen always smells bad to me," he said. "I don't think it really does, I think it's just an association that I have. It smells like rotten eggs. It's awful."

"Jump into the river again and wash that association away as you washed the shame away." I told him.

He rose to his feet and paused for a moment at the rock's edge.

"Get it really strongly in your mind, that bad smell. This is what you're being cleansed of. Let the river take it away."

He gathered himself a moment more, and then leaped into the water. I remained on the rock, and a few seconds later he emerged laughing.

"It's gone!" he exclaimed in delight.

I smiled at him as I reflected upon how much I loved this man, how privileged I was to be able to make a difference in his life.

We rested on the rock for a while, and then started back down stream. The trip was much easier than before, and on the last stretch we put snorkels on and swam down the river like fish. The current pulled us easily and we glided through the rocks, seeing their underwater curves flow by.

A few weeks later he called.

"I just wanted to tell you that the shame is gone," he said.

"Gone?" I asked, amazed.

"Gone. No more shame. Not once."

The Bust
2003 (age 49)

I. The News Breaks

I listened to the incoming message on the answering machine, wondering if I should pick it up.

"Call me as soon as you can," Ava said. "It's important."

I picked up the phone. "Hi, Ava. What's happening?"

"We got busted! Cops broke down the door. It was awful."

I felt my blood run cold, and I sank into the chair. Paralysis set in. I was frozen and panicked.

"What happened?" I asked.

"I was just starting with a client. I still had my dress on. They broke down the door, seven of them with guns. They took him into a different room and questioned him for a while, and they questioned me. I remembered to say that I wanted to be silent and I want my lawyer, so they didn't ask me anything after that. After a couple of hours they let me go."

"That's good. You did well."

"I don't know what happened to Sally. She's not there. I don't know if she got arrested, or if she went home. The laundry's still there, and she was going to take it, so I don't know what's going on."

"I'll try to find out. Thanks for calling me, Ava."

I hung up the phone, and went to find Peter. "They busted the place tonight."

He looked at me in concern. "Oh, no! Is there anything I can do?"

"Yes, you can shred documents for me." I gave him all my papers about scheduling, accounting, anything I could find about the business. "I have to try to find out what happened to Sally."

Sally was my best friend and I was worried about her. I called every number I had for her, with no answer. Finally, I tried her boyfriend's number.

"Have you seen Sally?" I asked him urgently.

"She got arrested tonight. She's in the police station now. She called me. They've had her in there for hours. I'm trying to get her out."

"Oh, god, how awful."

"Yes, well, I'll stay here until I get her out."

Reassured that someone was caring for Sally, I placed a call to a lawyer whom I had heard was good with defending sex workers. I explained the situation to him.

"Are you afraid that the women arrested might say that they were working for you?" he asked diplomatically.

"Yes, my name is on the lease of the apartment."

He gave me some brief instructions of what to do, and we set up an appointment to meet in person in a couple of days. He agreed to refer Sally and Ava to the appropriate lawyers. I felt relieved that he seemed so competent.

The next morning, I took my computer to a friend's house so that it would not be confiscated if they came to my house with a search warrant. I used his phone to call the other women who worked for me to tell them not to come to work. As I talked with each one, I felt the loss of the dream more and more keenly. Such high hopes I had held, and they were all dashed to bits in an instant.

II. The Temple Begins

I walked through the large rambling house with Jay, looking at it for the first time. He was Karen's lover, my former madam. In the months since I had worked for her, we had remained friends. Fascinated by her work, he had decided that he wanted to be a part of it. She introduced us, and we worked out an arrangement in which he would rent the house and fund the operation, and I would manage the employees. We agreed that to the employees, he would just be Sam the handyman, for his legal protection, and to make me the only one in authority. I knew well the potential for "Mommy and Daddy" projections from the women, and the games that could ensue.

Although I did not know him well yet, I had enjoyed our interactions. He was witty and charming, and he made business meetings fun. We had a very harmonious partnership so far, and we shared a common spiritual orientation. He had been a yoga teacher in the late 70's, and had practiced meditation for many years. We had spent a pleasant hour in the park doing yoga in between looking at houses. He was a handsome man, with dark skin and hair, hazel eyes, and the body of a former yogi, and there was some sexual tension between us. Neither of us wanted to act upon it for fear of spoiling our business partnership, so mostly it was unspoken, and expressed in wild flirting that we knew wouldn't go anywhere. I could tell that he was a resourceful and intelligent man. He had spent months looking for the perfect place.

The forest green carpet was luxurious. The layout of the house was ideal for what I wanted. There were four bedrooms, and a separate space for the women workers to rest and visit with each other between clients. I felt the potential of the temple there. I didn't know yet who would work there, but I knew that this was my chance to create a temple like never before, at least, not in the last 5000 years. This was the place to house a temple of the sacred prostitute.

"I like it, Jay. I think this is it."

III. Fear Continues

The second morning after the bust, I was doing yoga at my home as usual. Sitting in front of my altar, I had the thought, "If I go to prison, I can teach the other inmates yoga."

There were three potential charges that I was facing: pimping, pandering, and conspiracy. Pimping is deriving income from someone else's prostitution. Pandering is enticing someone into prostitution. Each of those "crimes" carries a mandatory three-year state prison sentence. Conspiracy is more variable, up to the judge's discretion.

I broke down into sobs, fearing for my freedom. I wondered how such holy work as I was doing could be so disapproved of that it was illegal. It didn't seem right.

IV. Growing the Temple

We opened for business on Valentine's Day. Three of us women were there -- Kelly, Roxanne, and myself. Kelly was a tall young woman, perhaps twenty-three years old, a mix of Caucasian and African-American. She had lots of small long blond braids, creamy skin, and an innocent girlish voice. Roxanne was in her late thirties, with wild auburn hair and a long slender body. We were idle for most of the day, since not many people knew we were there yet, so we chatted and got to know each other. I found that Kelly had been in the sex business since she was seventeen. She had been abandoned by her mother, and ended up on the streets. She didn't tell any details of that time, but I got the impression that it was traumatic. She had shifted from doing full service (intercourse) to only doing sensual massage. Roxanne seemed very anxious to please, and a little nervous. She really wanted to do things right. It was unusual for me to feel like a boss, but I could tell that she was putting me into that role.

Finally, one of my favorite clients called, and I did a session with him. We had fun and passion together. It felt fitting that the first session in the new temple be mine, and with a client that I really enjoyed.

The business grew rapidly. The women who worked for me told their friends about the place, and soon I had a waiting list of people who wanted to work there. I only accepted women who had a consciousness of sacred sexuality, and who understood the power of using sexual energy for healing and transformation. I worked hard on establishing procedures and systems, so that things flowed smoothly. Clients discovered us quickly, and soon we were seeing twelve or more men per day, with three women working each day. The sacred space that we were creating drew them in.

I began each morning sitting in a circle with the women working that day. I led them in a meditation.

"Feel your root growing deep into the earth, drawing up the earth's energy with each inhale, and sinking the root deeper with each exhale. Allow the earth energy to move up your spine to your crown, and open your crown to Spirit. Let the top of your head be like a flower, blossoming open. Invoke the priestess energy. Ask for the energy of the sacred prostitute to enter you and inspire your actions today."

Each woman would then say her intentions for the day, and light a candle on the altar to empower that.

"I want to bring light to each man that I see, and also to myself."

"I want to honor myself and my boundaries, and speak up when I need to."

"I want to have fun, and help all the men I see have fun too."

"I want to make a lot of money." We all chuckled.

I organized trainings for the women to take. The first one was about legal issues of the business. A lawyer came in and spent a day teaching us about the laws, how the police do things, and what to do if we were arrested. It was frightening to all of us.

"Let's put a dome of protection around this place, surrounding it with white light. Only that which is of our highest good may enter here." I felt it was important to balance the fear engendered by learning about the laws.

Next was a lesson in ergonomics. A woman who had been a masseuse for fifteen years taught us ways of using our bodies to help keep them pain-free. Repetitive motion injuries to the hands are common to masseuses.

I taught another session on grounding, protecting energetically, and clearing energy, all useful tools for the work.

The place began to feel even more like a temple, where young women were learning the arts of the priestess.

V. The Visit to the Lawyer

He was a knight ready to do battle, a high-testosterone man with high-strung assertiveness that could easily go into aggression. Just the kind of person I needed to protect me. Jay and I sat in his office, nervous and on edge.

"Do you have any enemies?" he asked. "Any former employees, or wives of clients? That's usually how this happens. The police aren't usually interested unless there's a complaint. So somebody must have complained."

"No, I can't think of anybody. I did fire a few people, but they all took it really well. Some of them even thanked me for it."

"What about Sally? Do you trust her?"

"She's my best friend, and she has been for years. I totally trust her."

"Be really careful with her. They could make a deal with her to drop her charges in exchange for her ratting you out. Don't talk to her about this case."

My belly clenched in dread. Not talk about this to my best friend? How could I do that?

"OK, if you say so. I won't."

VI. Upsets in the Temple

Within a month after we opened, it was clear that some of the women were not appropriate for the place.

"I don't want to work with Roxanne. She's really strange. She's ok when you are around, but when you're not she's awful. The other day while I had a client she got upset about something, and started doing some kind of primal scream in the living room."

"Yikes! I'll talk to her."

First I consulted with Karen. She had offered to help me with advice when I needed it, and I knew that she was levelheaded and experienced.

"Be very careful if you fire someone. You're vulnerable since it's an illegal business. If they decide they want revenge, all they have to do is call the police. Make them think that it's their idea."

I called Roxanne, and told her that some of the women she worked with had mentioned that she was having a hard time there.

"It's my PMS," she said. "I'm ok the first half of the month, but when I'm premenstrual, I lose it. I'm sorry."

"I'm sorry too. I just can't have that going on there. It's too disruptive."

"I understand. I don't blame you. Can I be on the substitute list for when I'm not premenstrual?"

"Yes, that would be fine," I said, knowing that I would never call her, but wanting to keep a good relationship for my own safety.

Marie was next. A tall slender woman with short blonde hair, she was working with me and also starting her own independent business. She had never worked in the sex industry before, and every time I was around her, she sucked me dry for information. Then she began to miss work. Her back went out, she was sick. The missed days accumulated.

I called her to check in. "Marie, sometimes your body is speaking to you when you have problems like this. Are you sure that you really want to be working for me, or do you just want to be on your own?"

"I think I really want to be on my own."

"Then I bless you in doing that. I don't want you here if you don't want to be here. Please don't stay out of any obligation to me. I release you from that."

"Really? Oh, thanks!"

I breathed a sigh of relief. Yes, make them think it was their idea. I wouldn't have to deal with her schedule upsets and grasping energy any longer.

Then came Olivia. A tall voluptuous African-American woman in her late thirties, she was Kelly's aunt and had helped raise her. Kelly had gotten her a job there with me. She was not doing well, seeing only one or sometimes no clients in a day.

"Let's see how this goes for a week or two," I suggested to her. "I like you, but this is wasting your time and mine."

She agreed, and evidently decided that it was not worth her while, because she never came back.

One Saturday morning, I got a call from Kelly. "I'm not going to be back to work on Monday, or after that. I'm moving to Montana. I'm on the plane now."

"You're giving me two days notice?" I asked with some irritation. "That's not much."

"I know, I'm sorry. I just decided now."

"Well, I guess there's nothing I can do about it. Good luck with everything."

Two weeks later, she called me again. "I'm back. I decided not to move after all. Can I have my job back?"

I had not found a replacement yet, so I said that she could work on a temporary basis until I found someone. She was quite responsible for a couple of weeks, so I offered her the position again, on the condition that she commit to stay there for six months. She agreed, and began working regularly.

VII. Sally's Ordeal

I met Sally for lunch after the visit to the lawyer. I was nervous because of his warnings, but also concerned about how she was after her arrest.

"It was my last day of work before I quit to go to Brazil," she began. "It was a really slow day. I didn't see anybody that day until the guy that I think was an undercover cop. He told me that it was his birthday, and he was treating himself. He said he had never done this before and he didn't know what to expect. He didn't take his underwear off. I asked him if he wanted to, but he didn't."

"My lawyer said cops often don't take off their underwear," I confirmed.

"So he just kept acting kind of shy and confused. I got a little uneasy, and at one point I got off the table and put all his stuff in the closet – glasses, cell phone, watch. I closed the door, just like you said."

Often undercover police come into a session with hidden tape recorders. I had taught the women to put all their client's clothes into the closet and close the door so that any recording would be thwarted.

"I was trying to be nice to him. I asked him if he wanted to take his underwear off again, and he asked me what would I do if he did. I screwed up here; I said I would pleasure him. He asked me what that meant, and I said that I would stroke him. Then he asked me if he had to pay extra for that or was it included in the session, and I said it was included."

My heart sank, both for her and for myself. She had admitted that she would take money for sexual services, which is all that was needed to convict her. If she was convicted of prostitution, then I could be convicted of pimping and pandering.

"Oh, honey, I hope it all turns out ok for you," I said with concern. "This is so awful. What happened next?"

"So then he left and I was taking a shower. I heard a sound at the door, so I wrapped a towel around me and went to see what was happening. Before I could get there, they broke down the door. There were eight cops, with their guns pointed at me, as I stood there with my hair dripping."

"Talk about overkill! There were seven with Ava. Fifteen cops altogether for two unarmed women."

"Then they took me to the police station and held me for hours. It was about 2 AM by the time they let me go. It was terrible in there."

I hugged her. "I'm so sorry you had to go through that. If there's anything I can do to help, please let me know."

"OK," she hugged me back.

"My lawyer said that I shouldn't talk about the case with you," I said, hating that I had to be suspicious of her.

"That's fine," she said. "I'd rather talk about other things anyway. I found a home for my dog while I go to Brazil."

VIII. *Good Times in the Temple*

The rooms where the women stayed when not with a client were the central part of the temple. A large kitchen adjoined an area that we had furnished with a sofa and a desk. There was always a lot of activity here, with women coming and going in between sessions, often in various stages of undress.

One day, I was working with Sally and Joey. The two of them had become very close. Sally had realized that she had had an abortion the year that Joey was born, so Joey was like her daughter as well as her friend. They were a study in contrasts, Sally tall and blonde, with long legs and beautiful blue eyes, and Joey short and curvy, with short dark hair and dramatic brown eyes, especially when she had her exotic eyeliner on.

I walked into the rest area, wearing an ivory satin robe with nothing underneath. My hair was tangled and my face was flushed. Sally and Joey were roughhousing with each other.

"I'm being a Rottweiler!" Sally exclaimed, grabbing Joey around the waist and shaking her. "Arf! Arf!"

"Grrr!" Joey growled back. They scampered across the room towards me, laughing and playing.

I smiled at them. "That was such a fun session!" I enthused. "He was a real sweetheart. I liked him a lot."

Sally disengaged from Joey and turned to me. "Woof! Woof!" She grabbed me and picked me up, swinging me around. I shrieked in delight.

As she put me down again, the three of us came together in a hug.

"I love it here!" Joey said. "It's so much fun."

Chloe came walking into the break room. She was a belly dancer in her early forties, with long curly dark hair and hazel eyes. She dressed dramatically, with lots of arm bangles, scarves, and bells around her ankles.

"That man was challenging. He needed to learn about touching with an open hand, not grasping for my energy."

"What a beautiful way to say that," I answered. "I know just what you mean. I bet you were able to teach him a lot."

"I hope so. It was kind of draining."

"Have you cleared your energy?" I reminded her.

"Oh, thanks, I need to do that."

Jay was fixing a broken doorjamb, kneeling on the floor. I walked up behind him, and whispered in his ear, "Under these jeans, I'm wearing a black lace thong and black thigh-high stockings."

I walked away laughing as he moaned and dropped his head. "Uhhh . . . What was I doing?"

"Do you do prostate massage?" Rose asked. She was new in the business, and I was still training her. Her sweet heart-shaped face and sparkly dark eyes were enchanting.

"Yes, want me to tell you how?" I offered.

All heads rose, and the women there gathered. "I want to hear this too!"

I sat with them and explained how to do it. They listened raptly, and thanked me for teaching them.

IX. Personality Conflicts Surface

A few months after I rehired Kelly, I got phone calls from both Sally and Joey.

"Kelly is getting really hard to work with. She's different when you're around, but when you're not, she's really angry. She dumps a lot on us. It's really unpleasant. I think you should fire her."

What bad timing for a messy situation! I was moving, relocating to small town in the mountains, and trying to work out how I would run the business while only being there part-time. I was distracted and stressed. I let it go for a while, putting off dealing with it.

"I saw a woman here named Kelly last week," one of my clients said to me. "She was awful. She was almost rude. She acted like I was a monster. It felt terrible. I'll never see her again."

"I'm so sorry that happened. You're such a sweetheart; I don't know how she could have not liked you. I'm sure it was more about her than about you."

Obviously, something had to be done. I gave Kelly a call.

"Kelly, I've been getting complaints about your behavior from clients and from the other women. If you're acting like this, you're obviously not happy here. I'm concerned about you, and I want you to be in a situation that you like. I'm not sure that doing this work is serving you."

"Are you letting me go?" she asked abruptly.

"Uh, yes," I replied, a little shaken.

"I really need the work," she said. "I was planning to leave in another month to go on a trip. Can I just work until then?"

"Yes, that would be fine. But you need to straighten up. If I hear any more complaints, then you'll have to leave right away."

She agreed, and continued to work. Joey called me about a week later.

"I'm feeling sorry for Kelly now. I've been talking to her a lot. I think you firing her has reactivated her abandonment issues about her mother." Joey had a master's degree in social work. "I'm sorry I asked you to fire her."

I rolled my eyes. "Now she's sorry!" I thought to myself. "This job is more trouble than it's worth sometimes."

"I'll talk to her," I promised.

I called Kelly several times but she never returned my calls. About a week later, she didn't show up to work, and she never came back again.

X. *Trouble Brews*

I had taken a brief vacation, about nine months into our time in the temple. I insisted that all the employees take regular time off to recharge, and I tried to set the example myself. Driving back from the airport, I got a call from Jay. "We got an anonymous letter today from a neighbor. It was addressed to 'sex employe'. They spelled it with just one 'e' at the end. It says to take our sex business out of the neighborhood."

"Oh, no!" I cried.

"It also said that whoever it was had written another letter to the landlord."

"Uh, oh, that could be bad."

"I've called him and told him that I'm having some disputes with my ex-wife and she's getting very unreasonable. I told him that she's writing letters accusing me of all sorts of things."

One of his strengths for this business was in inventing compelling stories for landlords, utility companies, and whoever else needed to be deceived. I had no practice in lying, and I was awful at it. I understood the need for it in running an illegal business, but I had no aptitude. I was grateful that he did.

"I told the women to go home," he said. "They are scared."

"I'll give them a call."

The next three weeks were spent looking for another place, packing, and trying to stay in contact with the women, letting them know that we were doing all that we could to get back into operation soon. Jay found another house, but it was only two bedrooms. The location was ideal, so we took it anyway, and I had to cut back the staff. Some difficult decisions were required about whom to let go, and telling them was hard. Most were philosophical about it, and understood the position that I was in.

As we were packing, Jay seemed despondent. I asked him what was wrong.

"Karen dumped me," he replied.

I gave him a hug. "Oh, dear, you've got a lot going on at once. I'm so sorry. Anything I can do?"

"A blow job would probably be helpful," he joked with me. We laughed together, feeling ease in our connection.

The house was a bright yellow-orange color, built in the 1920's. It was lovely, but had been neglected and was in disrepair. Jay spent many hours repairing things. One day, I put my hand on the doorknob to open it, and it came off in my hand. I called Jay.

"Hello, I'm calling you from the Rotting Pumpkin. The doorknob just came off."

He laughed with me.

139

Things settled down again, and operations went back to normal. After about two months, I went out of town again for another vacation. Jay also went away at the same time. Back in town but not yet back to work, we met at the house to catch up. He was opening the mail as we chatted. Suddenly he cried out, "Oh, no! Not again!"

He held out a letter from the city government. In it, they said that they knew that we were operating an illegal massage business, that it was run by a woman named Selena, and that the women advertised on an adult entertainment website. It advised us to cease and desist, with a copy of the letter going to the vice department.

"I can't believe it!" I sighed. "So soon! What's going on?"

"I hate to say it, but I believe that someone is out to get you. They mentioned your name."

"How could anyone know my name? Would it be the land-lady? Did she hear it?" I asked anxiously.

"I don't know. But I do know we have to get out of here."

The next weeks were a nightmare. Again looking for a place, again packing, again trying to keep the staff together and op-timistic. Jay and I began feeling the stress. I was just entering menopause, and I was having twenty to thirty hot flashes a day. He came down with a cold, but refused to go home and rest.

In short order we found another place. I didn't like it, but it was the best we could find in such a short time. If we delayed too long, the women would have to go elsewhere to work, so we needed to come up with something soon.

We found two boxy, depressing apartments side by side. They were dark and dank, and smelled like mold. The women were not happy.

"It's only temporary," I assured them in a meeting. "I'm continuing to look for a better place. This is just so you can get back to work."

They grumbled but accepted it. Routine asserted itself again, and things became calm. Fatigued from two months of stress, I decided to take another vacation. While out camping by myself in the desert, I extended my trip another week. I had been back a day, still at my mountain home, when I got the call from Ava that we had been busted.

XI. The Temple Collapses

"What are we going to do?" Jay asked.

"I can't do this anymore. This has gotten too serious," I said in despair. "They just keep coming after us."

"I think you're right," he agreed.

"I just wanted to create a beautiful temple and do holy work," I sobbed. "What is so wrong with that? Why did this happen?"

He put his arms around me. "We did create a beautiful temple. It was great. And its time is over now."

Weeks went by and I spent time at home because I was afraid to advertise for doing massage again for fear of arrest. Sally's legal case dragged on. At last, I got a call from my lawyer's secretary.

"We got a copy of the police report. Do you want me to fax you a copy?"

I grabbed each page as it came out of the machine, eagerly reading it to find some clue of what had happened, who was responsible. Buried deep in the report was the answer. There was a copy of an anonymous letter sent to the police. It detailed the place where we worked, the names of all the women, with copies of photos from their ads, the fact that a woman named Selena ran the place, and that a man named Sam might be a partner. The letter was full of misspellings and grammatical errors.

"Sam! No one knows about Sam but the women! Oh, my god! It was one of the employees after all!" My mind raced. "Who could it have been? They can't spell --somebody who didn't get much of an education. Someone who hates me. . . Kelly! It was Kelly."

I grabbed my pendulum, a divination tool, for confirmation. It arced in the yes direction.

XII. Kelly

I was concerned for their safety, so I called many of the women who had worked for me, telling them of my suspicion that it had been Kelly who had sent the letters.

After warning the women, I dropped out from that world. I moved my work to a different city, and disappeared from everyone's lives except for Sally and Jay. I was too afraid to stay there, and I didn't know whom to trust. Even someone well-meaning might let some information about me slip to the wrong person, so I took no chances.

After our business dissolved, Jay and I had dinner one night at our favorite restaurant, where we used to have our business meetings. He walked me to my car in the rainy night, and we stopped on the sidewalk. He reached down and kissed me. I met his kiss with my own.

Several years later, Sally called me.

"I ran into Kelly the other day. She said that she never wrote those letters. She feels really bad that you told everyone that she did. She'd like you to call her."

Nervous, I gave her a call. I still was not sure what was true and what was not, but I knew that I didn't want her as an enemy.

"Kelly, I want to apologize to you." I said sincerely. "When I fired you, I was really stressed and distracted by moving. I regret that I acted so hastily. I should have been more understanding, and just given you a warning. I'm really sorry."

"Yes, it was hard then. I felt like you just kicked me out. It was awful. But I want you to know that I would never do anything like writing those letters."

Playing along, I said, "I'm sorry for thinking that you did. Everything pointed to you, so I just assumed. I'm sorry if that hurt you."

She accepted my apology, and we hung up in harmony.

I will never know who wrote those letters. Was it Kelly? Or Olivia? Or someone else whom I didn't even suspect? The mystery will never be solved.

Ultimately, it was not really about Kelly at all. It was bigger than that. The forces that disrupt the expression of the feminine were at work. The mother that abandoned, the young girl on the street, the toppling of the temple – all were a result of the attitude of dishonor toward the goddess. Thousands of years of patriarchy have created an environment where there is a split between feminine and masculine, earth and heaven, sexuality and the sacred. The healing forces of sexuality are despised and reviled.

Sitting in Karen's kitchen, a few months after the bust, I began to cry as I talked to her.

"It was so beautiful, what I was beginning to create. I had such hopes for a place of beauty and healing. It had such potential. And it was squashed, just like that. One person could bring it all down, just because it's illegal. It's not right. It was a place that served – the clients and the women who worked there. It was a place of goodness."

She smiled at me. "You didn't fail, and I didn't either. All those women that worked for you and for me – and there were a lot – they will never accept anything less now. They have learned that they have a right to work in a place full of dignity and safety. This area will never be the same for sex workers because they will not accept it."

Even though my personal dream of a temple was dashed, the times are changing. The sacred prostitute is becoming more accepted. It may take a while, but She is unstoppable now. The tide has turned. The priestess is returning.

Epilogue
2008 (age 54)

Here is an update on what has happened with the people in this book since the bust.

Chapter 1 – The Gateway

Initiation
In the past couple of years, this man has become extremely interested in personal growth. He has a morning practice of reading inspirational books and listening to CD's. He is relating what he is learning to what I taught him about Tantra.

Opening
Sean has connected with a beautiful woman who is a natural Tantrika. They did a few sessions with me together, learning how to bring more Tantric energy into their lovemaking. They are very much in love.

Shaft of Light
Jeffrey has been in a relationship with a woman for about two years. They love each other very much. They have occasional issues, but they are normal ones. He is amazed that he has actually found a partner, as he thought he never would.

Chapter 2 – Beginnings

Bondage
Peter and I have transitioned from a lover relationship to being great friends and companions. (More about that in my next book.) We share rural property, and see each other daily.

On Your Knees

Jay and I ended our relationship after five years. We are still friends.

Chapter 3 – First Loves

Male Love

Mark married a woman and had two daughters. Years later, when his daughters were grown, he told his wife that he was gay and they divorced. He is in the challenging process of redefining his identity. I lost touch with Dave.

The Pickup

I saw Wade once after our divorce. He had another wife already, and they were acting out the same patterns that he and I had done. I never saw him again.

Bad Trip Leads to a Larger Trip

Matt and I live in different states now. We see each other occasionally, and when we do we have an instant connection. It is always as if no time has passed at all.

Newly a Virgin

I saw Travis a few times after our divorce. Each time we had less to say to each other, until I finally stopped calling him.

Chapter 4 – Tantra

Doing It Right

Paul has been a Tantra teacher for many years. When I last saw Andrew, several years ago, he had a partner and a daughter.

A Secret Revealed

Scott and Johanna are no longer a couple, but each of them still teaches Tantra.

Chapter 5 – Building the Temple

Sensual Massage
Karen still does sensual massage, working on her own. We are still friends. Lilah moved out of doing sensual massage into teaching Tantra privately.

Heart Energy
I lost touch with Dan when I had to change my name after the arrest. I've often wondered how he is.

The Bust
Sally is still my best friend. She lives in another state, but we talk frequently on the phone and visit when we can. The prostitution charges against her were dropped after almost a year of being in the court system, largely because the recording that the policeman made was garbled since she put his things in the closet.

Roxanne and Rose are still practicing sensual massage. Joey has become a sex educator. Chloe continues to belly dance and do private sessions in Tantra. Marie established her own sensual massage practice. I lost touch with Ava, Kelly and Olivia.

Glossary

Chakra: (Sanskrit: wheel). A whirling vortex of energy in the subtle body, mostly located along the spine. Different chakras have different attributes associated with them.

Chakra	Name	Location	Attributes
First	Root	Perineum	Grounding and survival
Second	Sex	Lower abdomen	Sexuality, sensuality, creativity
Third	Solar Plexus	Upper abdomen	Will, power, manifestation
Fourth	Heart	Center of chest	Love, compassion
Fifth	Throat	Throat, jaw	Communication
Sixth	Third eye	Center of forehead	Intuition, wisdom, visions
Seventh	Crown	Top of head	Connection with Spirit

Cord: A draining energetic connection. Different than a bond, which is not draining.

Ida: (Sanskrit: comfort). One of the three main energy pathways (nadis) in the body. Along with the pingala, the ida spirals around the sushumna, forming a pattern like the medical symbol, the caduceus. The ida is the feminine, lunar, yin energy. (See also pingala, sushumna.)

Kundalini: (Sanskrit: coiled.) The life force energy, often visualized as a serpent coiled sleeping in the pelvis. Once awakened, it can be directed through the body, moving through the nadis and affecting the chakras.

Lingam: (Sanskrit: wand of light.) Penis.

Nadi: (Sanskrit: channel). Energy pathway. See sushumna, ida, pingala.

Pingala: (Sanskrit: tawny). One of the three main energy pathways (nadis) in the body. Along with the ida, the pingala spirals around the sushumna, forming a pattern like the medical symbol, the caduceus. The pingala is the masculine, solar, yang energy. (See also ida, sushumna.)

Sacred spot: G spot. Considered the internal seat of the second chakra.

Sushumna: (Sanskrit). The main energy pathway that travels from the root chakra up the spine to the crown. It connects all the other chakras. (See also ida, pingala.)

Yoni: (Sanskrit: sacred space). Vagina.

Printed in Great Britain
by Amazon

65493212R00099